# THE HIDDEN TRUTH
# BEHIND BEAUTIFUL SMILES

## Zack Zaibak, MS, DDS

"Chicago's Premier Dentist"

Second Edition

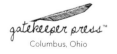
gatekeeper press™
Columbus, Ohio

iUniverse books may be ordered through booksellers or by contacting:

Gatekeeper Press
2167 Stringtown Rd, Suite 109
Grove City, OH 43123
www.GatekeeperPress.com

ISBN: 978-1-6629-1901-5 (sc)
ISBN: 978-1-4759-0654-7 (e)
ISBN 978-1-6629-1847-6 (hc)

Library of Congress Control Number: 2012937127

Printed in the United States of America

## contact

@Zaibak_Dentistry_Chicago

www.DrZaibak.com

1-708-802-9600

# CONTENTS

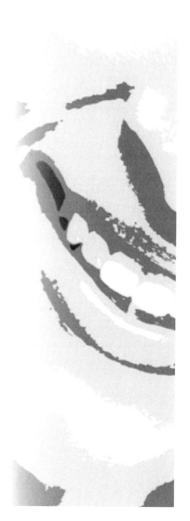

# ACKNOWLEDGMENTS

There are a number of people who've been very supportive in my life that I want to thank, beginning with my family.

I owe the deepest gratitude to my parents, who are the best I could ever hope for. They really were the perfect "team" to have on my side, always there when I needed them, always pushing me to be my best. More than anyone, they helped make me into who I am today.

I also want to thank my wonderful Grandma Sue Rafati, who offered me her generous love and support throughout my life.

My dynamic younger brother, Ed, was vitally involved in the creation of one of the first luxury green office spaces in the city. He's been active in numerous projects benefiting Chicago, appearing on local television, and rubbing elbows with the Daley family. I love Eddy dearly.

My lovely younger sister, Lina, is a wonderful person with a magical heart. She has excelled in her own medical career and is now a district supervisor for CVS Pharmacy. A caring, devoted professional, she always takes the time to educate her customers about the medications she dispenses.

My dearest wife, Aida—clearly it was fate that brought us together when she was chosen by her business school to represent Barcelona, Spain, at a convention in Chicago. Though she returned home after the convention, we stayed in touch. Once I completed dental school, I journeyed to Spain to meet up with her again. After all our years of "courtship," we moved forward rather quickly into marriage. The sweetest person in

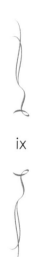

ix

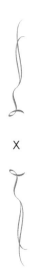

the world, Aida is a wonderful combination of intelligence and virtue. She always looks for the best in people. Outgoing and generous, she will give a friend the coat off her back. At the same time, she's no pushover. She loves to debate and is pretty skilled at getting what she wants—at least from me!

My love, you are the most beautiful and amazing woman in the world. I couldn't imagine a better person to share life with. You blessed us with our gorgeous daughter, Sarah, who's a constant source of joy and wonder.

I couldn't acknowledge my wife without also crediting her incredible parents. My father-in-law, Munir, was a very intimidating person when I met him. Physically large, with an intellect well known in his community, Munir owns a four-star hotel and carries himself in such a way that you feel you're talking to a president. He actually gave me a hard time at first, but I think he was testing me. My wife was his first daughter to be married, and I suppose I "took her away" from him. But I soon discovered that beneath his imposing exterior was a teddy bear with a heart of gold. He's since come to love me like a son, and now I have to laugh, "Why was I so nervous about this guy?"

My wife's mother, Maggie, is an all-out sweetheart. She's like a kid at heart and very playful. I am so very grateful to both of my wife's parents for producing such a wonderful daughter for me to share my life with.

I also want to thank my large extended family—my brother-in-law, two sisters-in-law, uncles, and aunts—for generously providing me encouragement and love. They have always made me feel very much at home with them, and I feel blessed to call them my family.

Additionally, I wholeheartedly wish to acknowledge my dental office employees. I am very fortunate to have such an amazing group of people working with me.

Helen is this wonderful spirit in our office, motherly and always seeing the good side of things.

I've known Aileen the longest of our employees, and she's been with me through thick and thin as we've met challenges, expanded, and improved.

Sue is the life of the practice—the jokester, always upbeat and smiling.

Salina is like the little sister in the office. The youngest of everyone, she's been with us since she was in high school. So she began with us essentially when she was a girl, and we've proudly watched her transform into a wonderful young woman.

Our hygienist, Angela, is the newest member of our team. She's my "ambassador"—the first person with whom patients have a "dental experience" at our office. Patients get comfortable with her as she expertly cleans their teeth, before they spend time with me. Angela is warm and fuzzy and a very hard worker. A highly positive person who takes her job seriously and performs her work enthusiastically, she's constantly looking for ways to improve her already impressive skills.

Thanks to all of you for your hard work, loyalty, and encouragement, and for delivering world-class patient-centered care to all of our remarkable clients.

I also wish to extend my thanks to Sohail Shafi, who has generously advised me in the

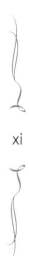

xi

best ways to run a thriving dental practice that is also highly successful and beneficial to patients.

Lastly, I want to acknowledge some of my friends. I've known my oldest and dearest friend, Bash (actually pronounced Bauche), since I was two years old. We've been through all kinds of adventures together. Being a pilot, he was the first person ever to fly me in a private four-seater plane. I actually feel bad for him, as I lost my breakfast in his plane that day. Like I said, we've been through a lot. We know everything about each other, to the point that there are times I can just look at him and know what he's thinking.

Dr. John, an eye doctor, has been like the big brother I always wanted. Our remarkable friendship curiously began with a boisterous handshake on the first day of my college ca-

reer. John quickly became and continues to be an inspiration to me—the type of man who is pure of heart and possesses kindness that you only read about.

Well known as one of Illinois' top immigration attorneys, Edwin played a vital role in my life, as it was through his efforts that my wife got permanent residency here. Now a close friend, Edwin is such an intelligent guy, you feel like you've learned something every time you speak with him.

Richie Lerias, DDS, is the first colleague I met in dental school. He is a wonderful person with a kind heart.

My friend Mario always gives 110 percent in everything he does, and he certainly serves as a good role model for me.

Jeff Korman, a close friend who graciously is helping to promote my book on a national level, and who also became a Snap-On Smile patient of mine.

I also want to thank John Eannace, a good friend who's been very supportive of my loved ones and family.

Constantly smiling, Tony is the life of the party who always speaks from his heart. It's always an incredible pleasure to spend time with him.

A great guy, my buddy Chris has soared above more than his share of challenges in life. Far beyond anyone else I know, Chris knows how to live life. He *embraces* it, living every day as if it is his best day on earth. Seeing how much fun one person can have motivates me even more to create that in my own life and my own family.

I am honored to count them all as my closest friends.

—Zack Zaibak

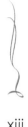

# INTRODUCTION

My journey into dentistry began when I was a boy. My parents had always pushed my brother, my sister, and me, molding us into successful adults. They encouraged each of us to take a different direction, based on our personalities. They wanted my sister to be a pharmacist and me to be a dentist, and in both cases they got their wish. They hoped my brother would become an attorney, though he became a businessman instead.

They chose dentistry for me because, as a child, I was always working with very small objects—opening up video games, assembling things. I can still remember my dad saying from the time I was very young, "You are really good with your hands." He himself used to be a jeweler, working delicately with small precious materials. One might say it was in the genes. So, from the time I was young, my father figured that I would be either a dentist or a plastic surgeon.

Perhaps the deciding factor was that I was always telling people, "You have a beautiful smile." It might seem an unusual thing for a kid to say, but the truth was I was always attracted to people's smiles and faces. Dentistry, therefore, seemed a natural extension of this fascination. My parents also had friends who became dentists, and they saw the lifestyle and family life the profession could provide.

My father owned a small grocery store, where I would help out. Here I learned many valuable experiences about relating with the public. I saw firsthand how people responded depending on how you interacted with them. This would later influence how I would create my dental practice.

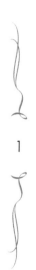

1

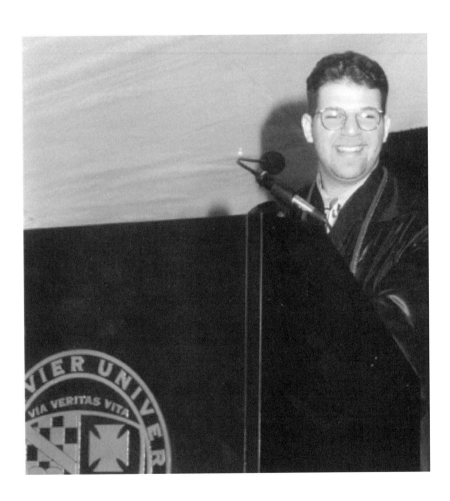

2

In college, a number of experiences furthered my quest into dentistry. First, a fellow classmate fell and broke her front tooth. Of those of us who were present, I was the only one who remained cool, suggesting, "Let's all just stay calm and have her stay where she is. I'll call her dentist and see what he can do for her." The dentist suggested I collect the broken tooth and place it in milk. Like some sort of dental paramedic, I quickly brought the tooth and my classmate over to him, and he took care of her.

Later, at Xavier University, I had a professor named Stanley Boyer who *almost* became a dentist himself. He had gone to dental school but for some reason chose to become a biology professor. In the class he was teaching (cadaver dissection), he was always pointing out the teeth, describing their names and functions. "This is the muscle for the lip, this for the jaw," I remember him saying. By the time the class was over, I knew more about the mouth and face than the rest of the body. Despite the unpleasant nature of the course—working with cadavers isn't everyone's cup of tea—it inspired me. Dentistry truly seemed to be my destiny. I graduated Xavier with a Bachelor of Science in biology and was named class valedictorian.

I've since had an award named after me, which is given every year to the graduating class valedictorian. It is called the Zack Zaibak, DDS, Outstanding Biologist Award.

From Xavier, I went straight to dental school at the prestigious University of Illinois at Chicago School of Dentistry, where I got my DDS (doctor of dental surgery) and a BSD (bachelor of science in dentistry), which allows me to teach dentistry if I choose. By the time I attended dental school, I pretty much knew what to expect, but I was sur-

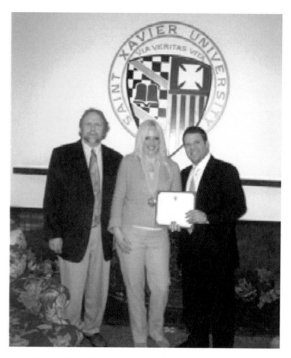

Me (on right) presenting my Outstanding Biologist Award to a recently honored valedictorian (middle)

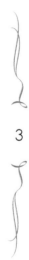

3

prised how much lab work we performed at this particular school. Normally a dentist simply takes molds and sizes and sends

4

them to the lab to manufacture crowns, dentures, and so on. However, we'd be making them ourselves! It was through this lab work that I learned firsthand a number of essential cosmetic dentistry skills, such as melting and casting gold and stacking porcelain on teeth. I'm grateful for the experience. Now if a crown were ever to fail, I would have a better understanding of why it happened. In my opinion, dentists who don't get this training are truly missing out. I also feel that dental school should be longer than it is. There's so much to learn. I wanted to be the best that I could be and to be fully prepared for my patients.

After completing dental school, I took the unusual step of taking an advanced general practice residency at Loyola Hospital. This residency gave me a couple of advantages before beginning my career. First, it put me into real-life situations where it was up to me

to handle whatever dental problems I might face, with no teachers to back me up. I did more dental surgeries in my residency than in four years of dental school. I was exposed to all kinds of complicated challenges, some of them extreme. People would come in needing teeth put back in after car accidents. It didn't matter if it was three in the morning—I had to be on my game. This also exposed me to the human side of dealing with patients—empathizing with their needs, hopes, and even fears about their teeth. I learned to work under pressure and to deal with complicated cases. In my practice today, I don't usually handle those "desperate" situations, but that experience has given me the confidence to handle any case that might walk into my office, and as a result, routine dental situations are now a breeze.

The other big advantage of doing a residency is that I rotated into other medical departments. For example, I did rotations in internal medicine, plastic surgery, and the ER. Hospital dentistry also gave me the opportunity to work on patients with all kinds of medical conditions and illnesses. These experiences exposed me to many kinds of medicine firsthand and helped me to become a *whole* doctor, not only a dentist. I learned about various conditions and how they might affect patients. For example, if a patient comes in with diabetes, I know what kinds of tests to administer before beginning treatment, and I'm aware that these patients might bleed more and take longer to heal. I also learned about medications and how they might interact with dental treatments. For instance, a patient taking medication that affects blood clotting might be prone to seizures during treatment. I can also detect oral pathologies, since one of my residency rotations was with the oncology department. Therefore, I'm more likely to

detect conditions like basal carcinoma. My patients might not see a dermatologist very often, but they do see me regularly, and in such a case I would be able to alert them to any potential issue so that a specialist could treat it early.

It's what I call "full-service dentistry," and it is the foundation for much of what I teach in this book.

## My Dental Spa

I think of my practice as a "dental spa." It has been specifically designed to relax patients who might otherwise be nervous going to the dentist. We have lounge chairs, sofas, and massage chairs in the waiting room. Even our dental exam chairs are massage chairs, lined with soft linen blankets and padded pillows. While in the chair, patients can watch television or listen to CDs of their

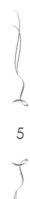

5

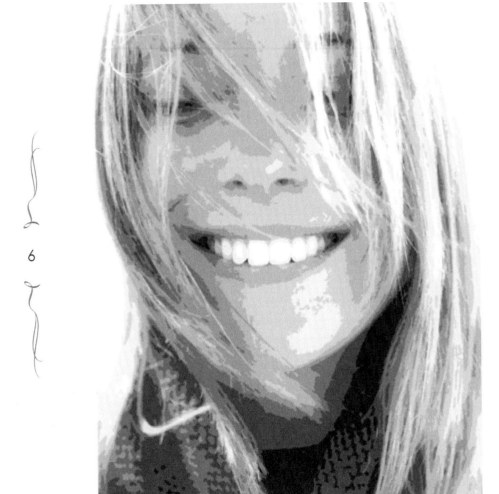

6

favorite music created especially for them. Once we have finished, we hand our patients warm face towels to refresh themselves. Our decor is also designed to be relaxing, with muted lighting, candles, and soft colors. We even have a large exotic fish aquarium, which many of our patients find relaxing. We offer extensive educational materials and videos, and we offer a variety of gourmet beverages, such as cappuccino and herbal teas. A visit to our clinic feels like a day at the spa. This helps our patients feel more comfortable coming here and melts away any fears. I've even had people say it makes them *want* to come to their dentist.

You might be thinking we cater to a high-end clientele. In fact, while we do neighbor a fairly affluent locale, we're actually located in a blue-collar area. In our opinion, everyone should be relaxed when visiting the dentist's office. The truth is people have to go to the dentist. They have to get their teeth cleaned. They may need to get a filling. So why not do it in the most pleasant way possible?

I treat my patients like family. When recommending any procedure, I always ask myself: would I recommend this procedure to my wife, my mother, or my dad? This policy comes from my father, who told me I should always treat people the way I want to be treated. This is especially important in a dentist's office, a place where trust is so important. Our goal is to make our patients feel secure, relaxed, and right at home. This way they are better able to express their concerns to me, and it ensures the patient–dentist relationship is a healthy one. I truly want my patients' time in my office to be a healing experience.

## The Passionate Dentist

Sometimes when I tell people that I'm a passionate dentist, they get the wrong idea. I'm not talking about an *amorous* dentist. I'm talking about someone who truly relishes what he does, every day. I love that I can help people. In addition to being passionate, I believe in being *compassionate* with my patients, treating them like my own family. This has earned their appreciation.

Some even call me "Doctor Z, the Magician." That's mostly because of the many smile transformations I perform using the latest dental procedures, such as Invisalign and Lumineers. A lot of my patients' friends and colleagues have done traditional veneers, and my patients have seen what their friends went through versus what they went through. My patients would say, "I had no

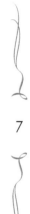

7

discomfort. My procedure was completed in two weeks, and I look fantastic!"

I love doing Lumineers. I love that people can change their lives in just two weeks. Creating a perfect smile in such a short time is amazing to me. Nothing compares to that incredible look on the patient's face when their case is done ... and the hug they give me. That feeling when someone new now believes 100 percent in my capabilities—it's the best feeling in the world, and it makes me want to keep doing better and better work. They're so satisfied with the results and the affect it has in their life that they refer their friends. It's an amazing chain of positive results that goes on and on.

Part of being a good cosmetic dentist is the ability to read your patient. Sometimes a patient will not elaborate on the kind of smile they want; but if they can't tell me what they

want, I can't deliver it to them. I may have one idea of what beauty looks like while they have another. So it's important that we agree before we start anything. Fortunately, I've developed a knack for getting information out of patients. I now know the correct questions to ask to learn exactly what will make them happy.

My real satisfaction comes when I see the changes their smile makeover has made in their life. They start to dress younger. They talk younger. They begin to take better care of the rest of their body—they go to the gym, they eat better, they lose weight. They start to get fewer cavities, because they take better care of their teeth now that they have a really nice smile worth protecting. They come in more often for checkups. A person who never smiled suddenly begins smiling broadly and talking more. They are more outgoing. You can feel the boost in their confidence.

I recently worked on a former Mrs. Illinois, America. She'd already won many competitions and had retired from competition. But after I put Lumineers on her teeth, she became more confident than ever. She's entering another pageant, for Mrs. Illinois, USA.

I had a young man come in, who was in his late twenties. His teeth had been pretty bad since he was a teenager. Some were crooked and misshapen, while others were simply discolored.

Somehow he was aware that they were hindering his life. I'm not sure if someone said something to him or he just deduced that on his own, but he told me that he hadn't been successful at dating, and at work he seemed to get passed by for promotions that went to less qualified people. So we talked and set

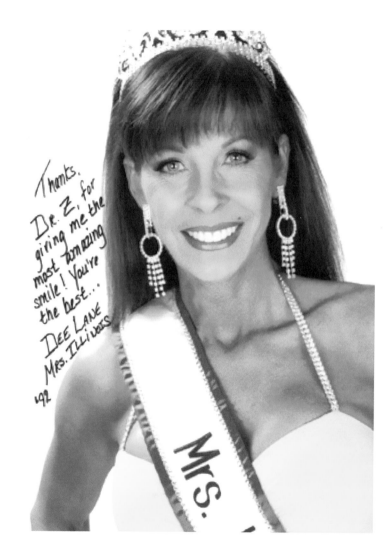

Thanks, Dr. Z, for giving me the most amazing smile! You're the best...
Dee Lane
Mrs. Illinois '12

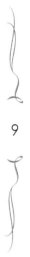

9

out a course of action to improve his smile. He was hesitant to pursue this, because he thought it would be too much hassle and too expensive. But he was committed, and it indeed turned out to be easier and cheaper than he had anticipated.

He had excellent results. By that, I don't just mean that his smile improved. It really did, but the results *in his life* were truly impressive. He said his new smile made him "smarter." It didn't, of course, but that's how he was *perceived*. He got a promotion three months after we completed our work. He's also been much more successful dating. He found that he didn't have to *try* so hard with women (which probably wasn't helping his cause in the first place). They seemed more at ease with him now. He wasn't sure if he was saying anything differently compared to before, but they seemed to be *listening* differently. Now, rather than hoping to get

*any* date, he could pursue women he was attracted to. Last time I spoke with him, he told me he had a serious girlfriend.

One of my patients had always wanted to move to Hawaii and create a life over there. She had very dark stains on her teeth from tetracycline antibiotics. She had tried many bleachings, but they remained gray.

Once I put Lumineers on her, her confidence jumped (pictures on facing page). She began doing the things she always wanted to do in life—including moving to Hawaii and getting a job over there!

I was surprised to see the sudden shift with this woman, but the truth is I had seen it happen numerous times. It's amazing how poor teeth can get in the way of dreams.

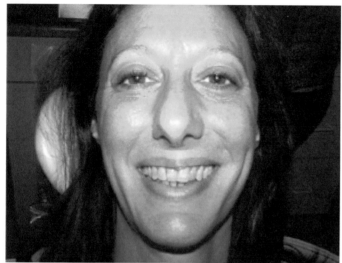

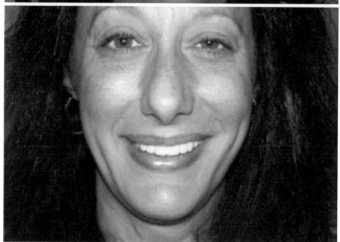

Interestingly, I also get a lot of women and men who are going through trouble in their relationships, who want a smile makeover to help them feel better about themselves. Soon, however, they find things start to improve with their significant other! They now have a nicer looking smile, which increases their self-confidence, and suddenly their loved one is more attracted to them and tries harder to make things work.

I recall one such patient who came to me. She had Lumineers put in, and six months later, I saw both her and her husband in my office acting all lovey-dovey. She came in to thank me for making her life better and for making her more attractive to her husband.

The improvements didn't stop with her mouth. Feeling better about herself, she began to take care of her hair, her makeup, and the way she dressed. But it started with

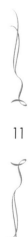

11

the improvement in her teeth. Her husband noticed not only her beautiful new smile, but that she was taking better care of herself, and he appreciated that she was going all out for him.

It's like I'm saving marriages, which only further proves that a great smile can really change your life.

I had a more extreme case where a patient came in having worn dentures for the last twenty-five years. She'd had all her teeth pulled when she was twenty years old while living in Russia. She was still an attractive woman. She pulled out her dentures and said, "I keep this in all the time. I've never even taken this out for my husband. He doesn't even know I have dentures! But I cannot stand this anymore. I feel very old."

That kind of story puts a tear in a guy's eye. Obviously the range of dental treatment for a person missing all their teeth is limited, and obviously whatever you do will be expensive. But when somebody is in such anguish over this, they will go to all ends to get what they want. So we did full-mouth implants on her, placing crowns and bridges over the implants. It was a lot of work, but it completely changed her life. She no longer has to lie to her husband and keep those dentures in all the time. Now she actually has teeth. He absolutely noticed her smile was better and whiter, and he loved it. He even came to my office himself and thanked me for working on his wife's teeth.

I have many autistic children as patients too. Something about autistic kids touches me. It's so tragic that we still misunderstand why they are the way they are. I donate free dental work to certain autistic organizations when I can, but one specific child stands out. I got a call from his father on a Sunday night after the boy fell. The father took him to the emergency room, but no one there wanted to help him.

So I decided to open up my practice late one night and see him. It was difficult, as autistic kids are very challenging to work with and require a lot of patience. But I was able to relieve the child's pain and fix his front tooth. I didn't charge them at all. Sometimes you just have to do things like this. I believe when you do a good deed, good karma comes back to you. In fact, there was even an article in the *Chicago Sun-Times* about my practice not so long ago about acts of kindness.

In addition to creating good karma, another core belief of mine is that I always need to be the absolute best that I can be. Always. Especially in my work.

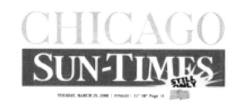

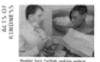

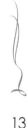

## *The Leading Edge of Dental Science*

Some people get to a certain point—in education or in how they conduct their business or even their life—and they stop. It's where they feel comfortable. It's familiar. They don't strive to change or improve themselves. But the world is always changing. Technology is always improving. It's moving so fast now that if you're not moving ahead by trying to change and improve, you're actually falling behind just by standing still.

13

But I've always made it my mission to stay on top of technology. If you consistently incorporate the newest technology into your practice, you're always going to be on top of things and passing along those benefits to your patients. It makes my patients want to come back to me, because they know I'm giving them the best that dentistry has to offer.

This is why I am constantly seeking additional education opportunities, accumulating over a thousand continuing education hours, not just the minimum number of hours required to keep my license current. In addition, I'm always reading up on new products available to dentists. If it fits with my practice and philosophy, I don't wait—I get it. I'm very happy to be the first on the block to have a new piece of technology.

This is particularly true with cosmetic dentistry. I take every course offered on Lumineers and Invisalign. They're always advancing the technology. I also take classes with an elite institute for cosmetic dentistry, called LVI. While there are many organizations out there teaching continuing education, this one is truly advanced, almost like a mini-residency in the latest cosmetic dentistry.

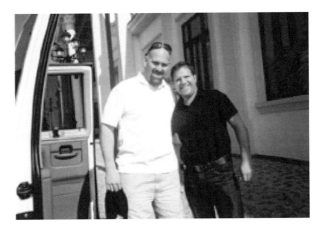

Meeting Boston Red Sox baseball legend Kevin Youkilis when Dr. Zaibak attended advance training at the American Academy of Cosmetic Dentistry Conference held at Harvard Dental School.

14

As a result of all that I strive to do, I've drawn a good deal of attention, both locally and nationally.

I've been featured in various publications, and for the last two years have been honored as one of the "Top Doctors" in *Chicago* magazine's "Best of the City" edition.

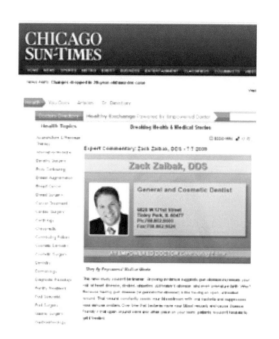

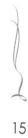

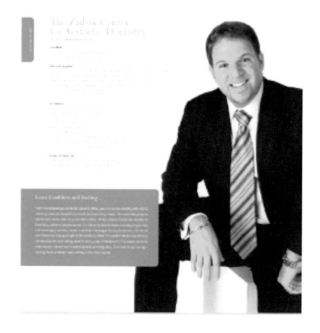

I was also asked by the *Chicago Sun-Times* newspaper to provide expert commentary in their health section for articles related to dentistry.

Additionally, for the last five years, the Consumers Research Council of America voted me one of America's top dentists.

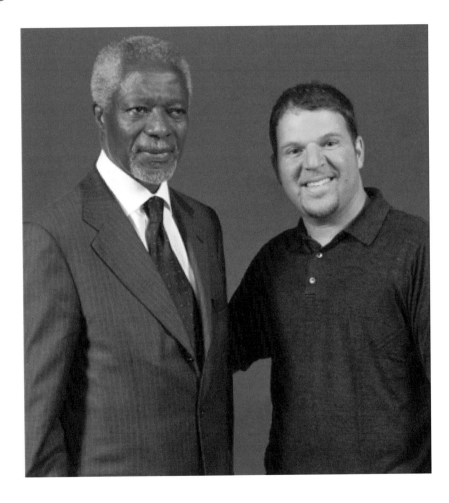

16

Plus, I have been interviewed on the local news in Chicago.

I also had the honor of meeting with the former secretary-general of the United Nations, Kofi Atta Annan.

We had a discussion about me becoming involved with Operation Smile, a children's medical charity organization that provides reconstructive surgery for children around the world born with facial deformities, such as cleft lip and cleft palate. He was especially interested in me because I had taken the advanced general practice hospital residency after completing dental school.

I've actually been involved with a number of charitable organizations. Not only can I be of service, you never know who you will meet.

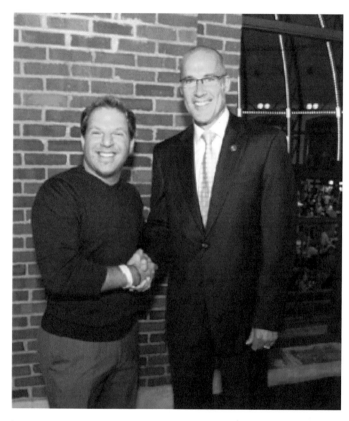

Spending time with Chicago Bulls John Paxson at a Taste of Nations Stop World Hunger event.

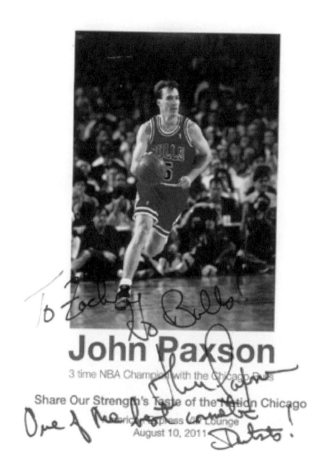

John's autographed poster calling Dr. Zaibak one of the best cosmetic dentists.

Being well-known locally has involved me in all kinds of organizations.

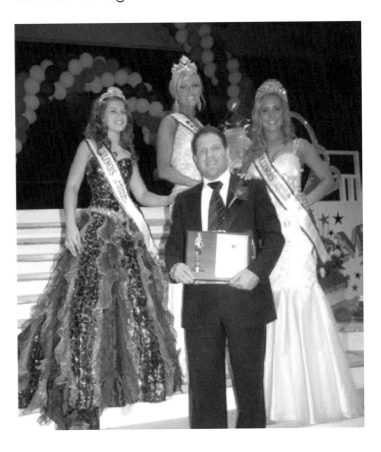

18

I was recently asked by the pageant committee to serve as a judge in the Mrs. Illinois America and Miss Teen Illinois America beauty pageants, because of my background as a cosmetic dentist involved in improving appearances.

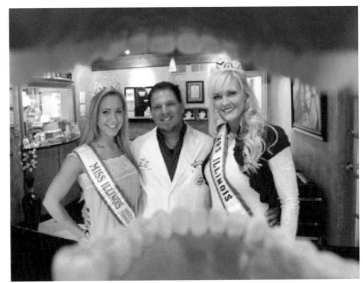

Over twenty contestants competed with just three chosen, based on their interview, looks, and smile. It was very difficult to choose among so many talented and beautiful women, but in the end, we knew we chose the right ones to represent our beloved state of Illinois. I can say the one thing that the winners have in common is a great smile, which will truly enhance their chances at the national competition. I also had the honor to treat the winners cosmetically by laser whitening their teeth, as an added award from the Zaibak Center for Dentistry.

I tell you all this not to pat myself on the back, although I will admit that with these awards and magazine articles coming my way, some other local dentists are asking how I am getting all this attention. I don't really have an answer for them, except that people get recognized when they are pas-

sionate about their field and about doing their best work.

Making myself and my dentistry better is what I love. It brings me immense satisfaction to be able to utilize my knowledge, skills, and passion to improve the appearance and the lives of my patients. I'd suggest to everyone to keep learning and improving. Not only will it make you better at whatever you do, it will keep you stimulated, involved, and ultimately happier.

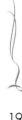
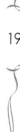

19

# CHAPTER 1

## HAPPINESS SHINES THROUGH YOUR SMILE

Happiness.

All our goals are just a means to achieving it, whether it's financial security, a big house, a satisfying career, fame, creating a wonderful loving family, helping your neighbor, or bettering mankind. Yet, despite people's success, many find this goal elusive. They have made money, raised families, and found love, but they haven't found the long-term happiness they expected. So what is missing? Sadly, what these people may be lacking is positive self-image.

For better or worse, first impressions are powerful. They can tell us if we'll trust someone, if we want to work with them, or if we are romantically attracted to them. This certain-ly applies to one's smile. Like someone with attractive, inviting eyes, someone with a beautiful smile is seen as personable and lik-able. If a person's teeth are dirty or crooked, we may form negative opinions of them before we even get to know them. In addition, these people will often go out of their way to avoid smiling, particularly when pictures are being taken. They may appear to scowl in pictures, or else they contort their mouths into a close-lipped smile that makes them look tense. They may be cheerful and warm on the inside, but because they never smile, the outside world never gets a window into this aspect of their being. On the other hand, a beautiful smile is a primal, universal symbol of health and vitality. An enthusiastic, joyous smile lights up a room like a lighthouse beacon. We've all experienced being in the company of someone who is in the bliss of true joy. It's wonderful. We feel like if we are around them, we can catch some of it

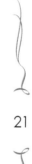

ourselves. Conversely, we know how draining it can be to be around someone who is always down or negative. Who would you rather spend time with?

In my experience with people of all socio-economic groups, having a healthy, attractive smile plays a vital role in one's happiness. Perhaps you think that's self-serving of me to say—but it's true. From a practical standpoint, great teeth will help you chew food better and allow you to derive greater enjoyment from eating. But that's not what I'm talking about here. I'm talking about the way people see themselves and the way they are seen by others. The truth is that in everyday life, people often size up one another based on how attractive they are. Numerous studies have proven that people tend to believe attractive people are more intelligent, trustworthy, skilled, dependable, fun, and simply more enjoyable

to be around. Naturally, one's appearance can't tell you that much about a person. However, consciously or unconsciously, appearance plays a significant role in how we form our opinions of others. Furthermore, we are acutely aware of the way we appear to others, and we act accordingly. Therefore, *people with unattractive smiles tend to smile less, while people with attractive smiles tend to smile more.* And people who smile more tend to be happier in life.

Some blessed people are born with perfectly white, perfectly straight, gleaming teeth. Yet that is rare. Most of us have smiles that are less than perfect to varying degrees. Ever since dentistry began, practitioners have been looking for ways to enhance their patients' smiles. Archaeologists have found crude braces consisting of metal bands connected by cat gut wires dating back more than two thousand years. However, it wasn't until the nineteenth century that orthodontics became a separate branch of dentistry. In recent years, methods to enhance one's smile have become far more sophisticated and numerous. Today, the best dentists practicing cosmetic dentistry are almost like artists. They can provide their patient with a variety of means to elevate their smile, matching it to that patient's face and personality.

## The "Chicago Smile"

In dentistry, people sometimes talk about that "Hollywood smile." This generally refers to those perfect smiles that so often flash across movie screens or billboards. Their teeth are aligned, bright white—perfect. Now they may not have started as perfect, and they almost undoubtedly didn't start in Hollywood either. Those smiles most likely came to Hollywood from someplace else.

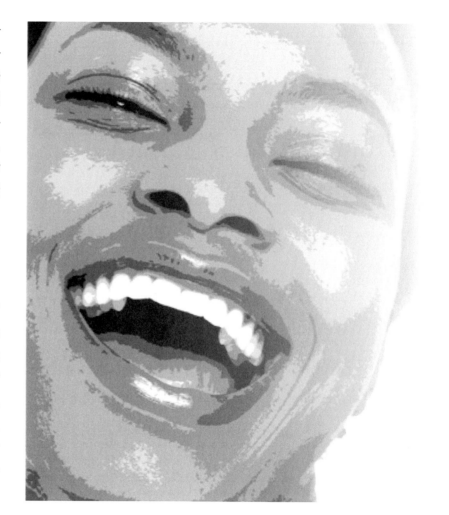

23

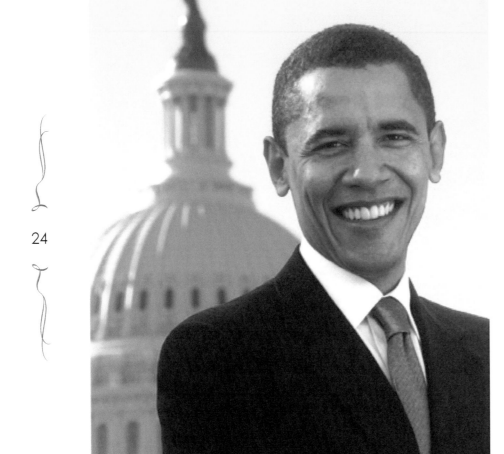

24

Many of them, including those of Jeremy Piven, David Schwimmer, Daryl Hannah, Vince Vaughn, Quincy Jones, John and Joan Cusack, Gary Sinise, and Virginia Madsen, came from my hometown of Chicago. Today, you can even see one of the smiles sitting in the Oval Office. While he's best known for his oratory skills, Barack Obama's smile certainly helped him secure the presidency. It is an engaging smile—masculine, strong, dependable, friendly, inviting, trustworthy. Another local smile that seems to be ever present belongs to the "First Lady of Chicago," Oprah Winfrey. Oprah's winning smile has helped propel a media empire.

Certainly all these people are very talented. Certainly they all have ambition. A good-looking smile never hurts either. However, Chicago isn't Hollywood. Hollywood is a fantasy world—unreachable, unattainable. Chicago, on the other hand, is a working city, full of regular people like you and me. While it has its share of glamour and celebrity, it is mainly comprised of real people, those like you, your family, your neighbors, your coworkers, your friends. Yet every day I see people walk out of my office with their new smiles, beaming with happiness and confidence, thanks to affordable procedures that weren't even possible twenty years ago. I like to call this smile the "Chicago smile."

## Symmetry Equals Beauty

People talk of "beautiful smiles." But the truth is there are different kinds of beautiful smiles, and different smiles that look better with different faces. A smile can even hint at what a person's personality might be like. For example, smiles can be masculine or feminine. Feminine smiles tend to be rounder, while a masculine smile is squarer. A good example

of a "strong, masculine smile" belongs to President Obama. While President Obama is clearly an accomplished adult, he can also exude a passionate hopefulness.

A smile should match the patient's facial structure and appearance. If the patient has an especially wide face, it's best to give their face a thinner appearance by making their teeth longer. If the patient has a very long face, it is best to give them a rounder appearance by making their teeth shorter and wider. The idea is to promote symmetry, because symmetry equals beauty. The shape of the individual teeth can be improved as well. Some patients want all their teeth to be even—straight across. Some smiles look better with squared teeth. Some look better with tapered teeth. Some look better with squared, tapered teeth. Other patients might want that youthful look with mamelons on the teeth—the little divots on

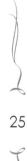

25

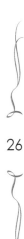

the edges of the teeth that you often see on children. Amazingly, all this can be created with today's advancements in cosmetic dentistry. A highly skilled dentist can truly be an artist.

In this book, I'll reveal state-of-the-art methods to help anyone look more beautiful. Many are fairly new, and they are easier and often less expensive than ever before.

### A Beautiful Smile Comes from Within

People who smile more tend to be happier, and when people are happier they start taking better care of themselves. This makes them even happier still, creating a positive feedback loop. This brings us to an important truth: while a gorgeous smile can certainly improve how we look, true happiness comes from within.

Now, there are as many paths to happiness as there are people traveling those paths. But there is a universal truth: our happiness is truly enhanced when we *feel better physically*. When our bodies are functioning well. When we are healthy. When we have an abundance of enthusiastic energy. Although it is possible, it is much harder to be cheerful if we don't feel good. I'm sure most of you have experienced this. Something isn't well in your body. Maybe something hurts. Even though it may be only in one area, your entire well-being is compromised.

People who are happy have an abundance of energy. I don't mean they're bouncing off the walls. But they do have plenty of vigor to pursue and *enjoy* the goals they set in life. Recall a time when you were especially tired or exhausted. Perhaps you didn't sleep well or hadn't been eating healthfully. If you can recall those times, you will likely

26

remember not feeling too happy. It's much harder to feel bliss when you are dragging your butt around. When we see people we admire, they not only have beaming, beautiful smiles, but they also exhibit plenty of enthusiasm, excitement, joy ...

Energy!

It's not just their external appearance that attracts us to them. It's also what's going on inside. In my field, I have patients come in who simply want to improve their smile. They want to look good and, of course, feel happy. But they are doing themselves a huge service when they also look beyond their smile—by maintaining a healthy body with high levels of vitality. In this book, I'll address not only oral hygiene but *whole body* care. After all, your smile is only the window to your temple. I'll speak of ways you can

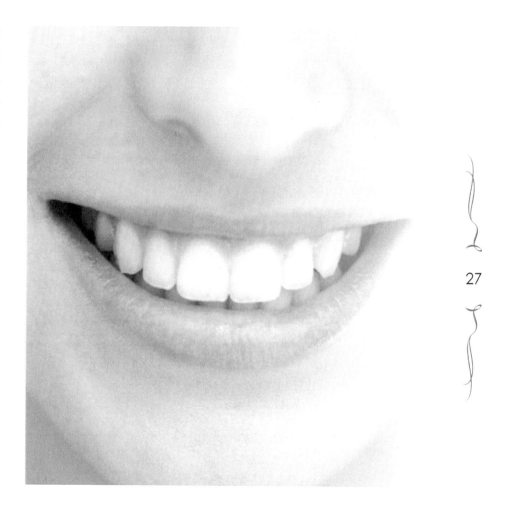

27

enhance your well-being, enhance your energy, and enhance your *happiness*.

In the first part of the book, we will talk about some revolutionary new procedures to enhance your smile and improve the function of your teeth: **Lumineers** and **Invisalign**. We will also talk about the latest advancements in teeth whitening, particularly the **Zoom 2** system. In the second part of the book, we will talk about how you can maintain a healthy-looking smile for the rest of your life. We will highlight the importance of regular dental checkups and give you useful tips on how to care for your teeth and gums at home. Your teeth are part of a larger, holistic system, and so it's important to be healthy overall in order to have a great smile. In the final chapter of the book, we will discuss ways to ensure that your body is getting everything it needs so that your great smile starts from the inside out.

# CHAPTER 2

## LUMINEERS—
## A MODERN MIRACLE

"Say cheese!"

We've all heard it, and for those of us with discolored, damaged, or crooked teeth, it can make us cringe as we imagine what we will look like when we flash a big, toothy smile. Because of this, we avoid smiling for pictures. Eventually this carries over into our day-to-day lives, and we find ourselves smiling less often. Soon, people stop smiling back at us, since they think we are unhappy with them. Our work relationships, friendships, and romantic lives suffer, and we may have the sense that we aren't living up to our potential. As a dentist, it saddens me to see people suffer this way, when today we offer treatment options that are painless, noninvasive, and affordable. That's why I have made it my life's goal to give beautiful smiles to as many people as possible.

Thanks to modern dentistry, no one needs to feel this way. There are many options for improving the appearance of one's teeth, including braces, contouring, and tooth whitening. However, undergoing some or all of these treatments may not be possible for some patients. Orthodontics may be too inconvenient for you at this time, or your teeth may be impossible to whiten because of tetracycline staining. Even if you are considering traditional porcelain veneers, perhaps you are (understandably) afraid of removing sensitive tooth structure, which is required before veneers are placed. Thankfully, there is now a process that can give you the smile you've always wanted in only two short visits to the dentist, with minimal pain, no an-

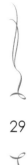

esthetic, and no removal of sensitive tooth structure: *Lumineers*.

Both Lumineers and veneers are thin shells of porcelain that are bonded to the front and top of the tooth. They can permanently close spaces between teeth, straighten misaligned teeth, and whiten dark teeth. For this reason, they have often been referred to as "instant braces." They can also improve the functionality of damaged teeth, particularly chipped teeth. I have always been a believer in non-aggressive, conservative dentistry. This is why I prefer Lumineers over traditional veneers in the vast majority of cases. Whereas veneers require the teeth to be ground down or shaved before they are applied—a sometimes painful process that removes sensitive tooth structure and requires anesthetic—the process of applying Lumineers is much less invasive. They are made from Cerinate porcelain, which is much thinner than the porcelain that traditional veneers are made from, and can be placed directly over the teeth without any grinding or shaving. They can even be placed over healthy crowns or bridgework (see chapter 5 for descriptions of these procedures) that may be old and need to be "refreshed."

I'm such a believer in this system that I've had advanced training in Lumineers. The Lumineers company recognizes me as a "Lumineers Smile Office," as we're one of their top offices, doing more Lumineers than anyone else in the state of Illinois. I have been invited to be on Fox, ABC, NBC, and WGN, to discuss this wondrous procedure (particularly its suitability for teenagers), and I've even been a guest speaker at dental conferences, as well as a teacher for the Lumineers company. In addition, I was recently interviewed by the premier Spanish-language media company in the United States, Univision, for a segment to inform the Spanish population about available treatments in cosmetic dentistry today, including Lumineers. I trust in the product so much, I have fitted my own mother with Lumineers. For all its benefits, it is truly a miracle of modern dentistry.

## Are Lumineers Right for Me?

Unfortunately, there is no simple answer to this question. This is a discussion that each patient must have with a Lumineers certified dentist. However, in my experience, the vast majority of patients are suitable candidates for the procedure. This includes patients with the following conditions:

- Spaces between teeth
- Stained teeth (in particular, tetracycline stained teeth, which cannot be treated with traditional whitening methods)
- Small teeth

- Uneven smile
- Chipped teeth
- Crowded teeth (however, this issue may prove more complicated; this can only determined by examination)

In short, the majority of minor cosmetic procedures can be addressed with Lumineers. Patients with an extremely bad bite (malocclusion) are not candidates for the procedure. In addition, you may not be a candidate if you have extremely large teeth or very large spaces between your teeth. This is because, in both of these cases, you are ultimately adding to the tooth structure, making the smile larger than it was. You'll end up with nice looking teeth, but they will be out of balance with the rest of your face. Such a patient may be a better candidate for traditional veneers, as they require the dentist to take away some existing tooth structure.

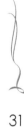

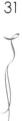

31

Trust me, a Lumineers certified dentist will never knowingly steer you in the wrong direction. We want you to look great. When you walk out of our office with a great smile, it makes you feel better, and that makes us feel better.

32

> *Beware of imitators. Only Lumineers use Cerinate porcelain, and only a Lumineers certified dentist can carry out the procedure.*

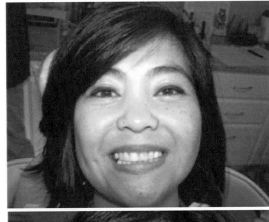

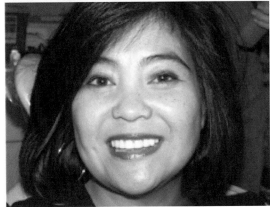

This patient already had crown and bridgework, but it was not that attractive. Rather than trim all that off, I placed Lumineers on top of them to improve appearance.

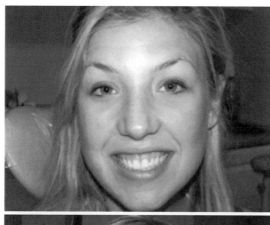

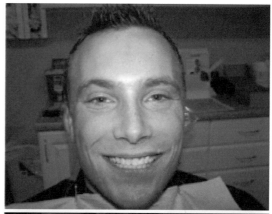

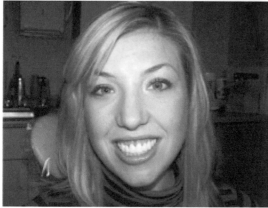

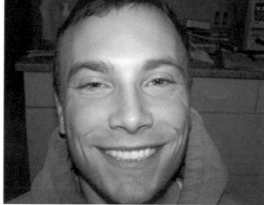

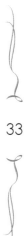

Lumineers were used to lengthen her upper teeth, along with some gum contouring to minimize the appearance of a gummy smile.

Though possessing a long-term fear of shots, Lumineers gave him a pain-free and pleasant way to reshape his teeth and keep them permanently white.

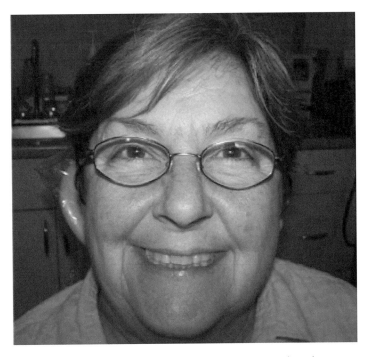

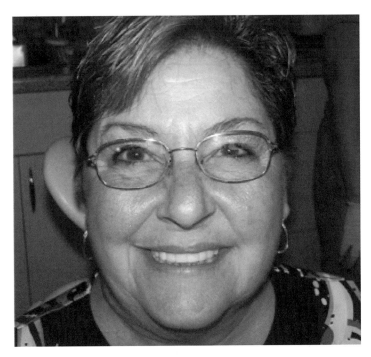

34

This patient had crowded, crooked, tetracycline-stained teeth that had worn down over the years. She was very unhappy with her appearance, and wanted the smile she had when she was twenty-one. However, she did not want braces.

We bleached her teeth and applied ten Lumineers on top. She was ecstatic with the results. She adopted a whole new outlook on life, dressing younger and becoming more active.

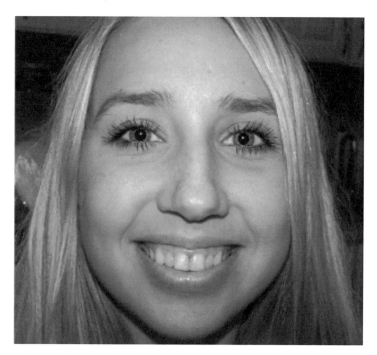

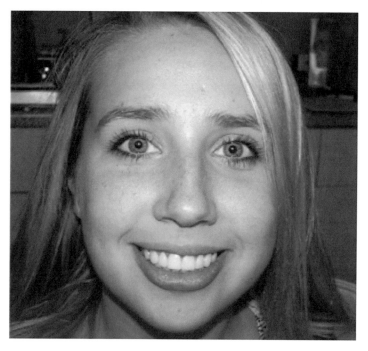

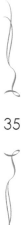

This young woman of Russian descent came in with badly decayed anterior teeth due to the poor living conditions where she grew up. She'd also gotten bad bonding, had stained teeth, and a gummy smile. When she came to the United States, the first thing she wanted to do was change her smile.

We performed a gummy smile lift, removed the existing bonding, bleached her teeth, and gave her ten Lumineers on the top. We literally made her American dream come true.

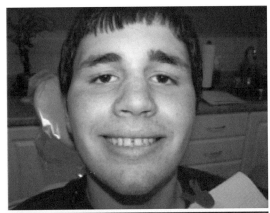

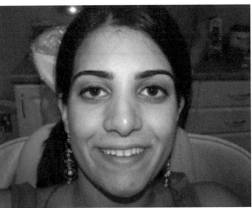

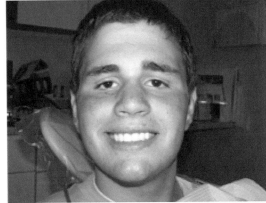

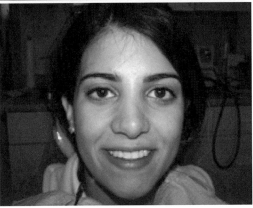

Lumineers closed gaps and whitened color. At a young age, this patient perfected his smile for an upcoming movie and continues working as an actor.

Lumineers were used to close gaps and change teeth color to permanent white, as well as increase size of teeth to proportionally match the size and shape of her face.

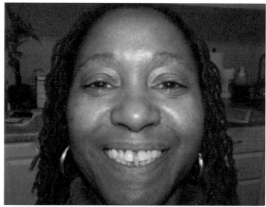

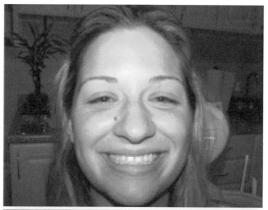

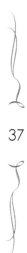

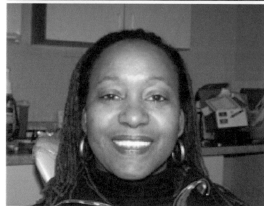

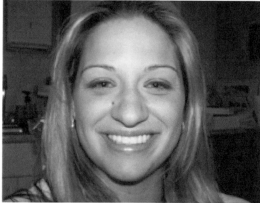

Patient wanted improvement in just two weeks without braces, in order to appear as a public speaker. We succeeded with Lumineers.

This massage therapist felt her teeth were too small. After Lumineers, she said, "This is the smile I always wanted!" Now she no longer hides in pictures. Even dyed her hair.

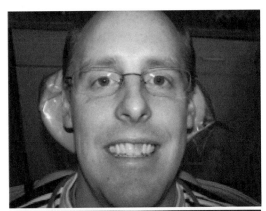

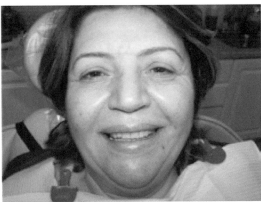

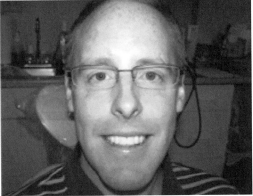

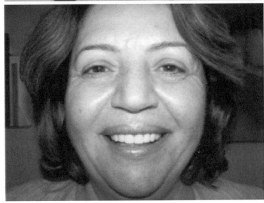

After a job loss due to the economy, he got nowhere with interviews. He thought improving his teeth would increase his job chances. After his smile makeover, every interviewer wanted him. "My best investment after my education!"

I so believe in Lumineers that I did them on my mother! She received ten Lumineers plus tooth whitening.

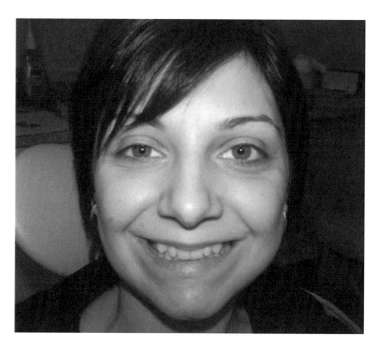

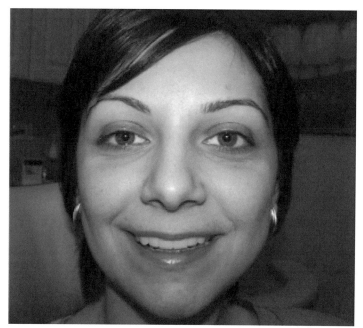

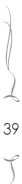

This patient, of Eastern European descent, had just gotten engaged and wanted a nicer smile for her wedding. She was unhappy with her protruding canines and with her teeth color. After two years of research, she still wasn't sure what to do. Then she saw me on a news feature and made the two-hour trip from her town to visit me.

After receiving ten Lumineers and teeth bleaching, she had the perfect smile to show off to her wedding guests. "The trip was worth every penny," she told me.

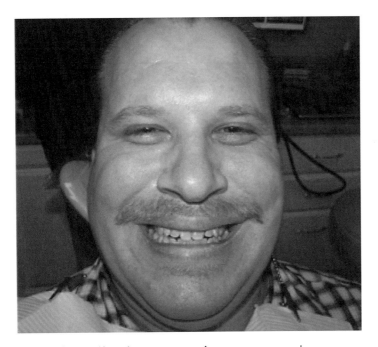

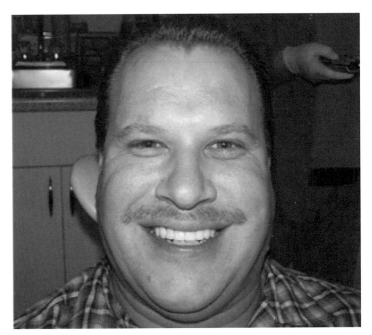

This patient grew up in an area where there was low fluoride in the water, so he had a lot of decay. He also had tetracycline-stained teeth, and he was unhappy with their color and shape.

We decided to give him twelve restorations, including Lumineers and ceramic crowns. He also got a gummy smile lift and whitening. For the first time in his life, he had white teeth rather than gray.

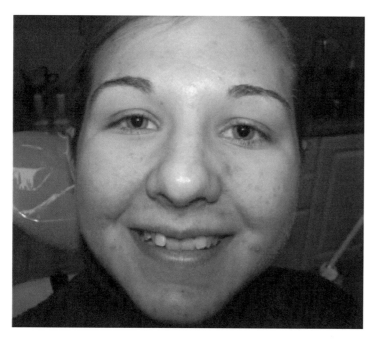

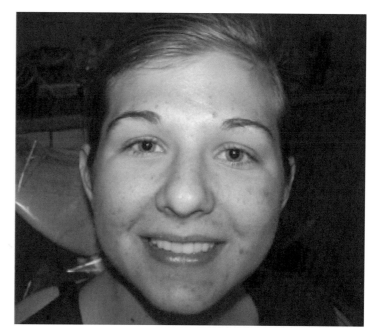

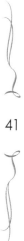

This was an extremely difficult case. This patient was very unhappy with her protruded laterals and teeth color. She didn't want Invisalign braces, and wanted a procedure that would not take more than a month.

We gave her ten Lumineers on top, bleached the bottoms, and did some gum contouring and crown work. She was so happy with the results that she just stood there with a mirror in her hand, crying. She couldn't believe the transformation.

### Getting Your Lumineers

As with any other cosmetic dentistry procedure, the first step to getting your Lumineers is *finding the right dentist*. You need to make sure that any office performing the procedure is a certified Lumineer Smile Office. This means the dentist has been certified as a Lumineer Certified Smile Dentist and has performed the procedure many times. This is critical. If your dentist is not a Lumineers Certified Smile Dentist, try to find another dentist in your area who is. An Internet search should help you locate qualified technicians in your area. (And don't forget to broaden your search to include nearby cities to which you would be willing to drive.) In addition, you'll want to ensure that whoever is performing your cosmetic dentistry has clean, modern, welcoming facilities. This is important when having any kind of dental work done. Don't be afraid to get two or three opinions before you make a final decision. Be sure you ask to see the cosmetic dentist's portfolio, containing before and after pictures and written testimonials, if possible.

Once you have found a Lumineers certified cosmetic dentist, you will have an initial consultation to review your case and assess whether you are a candidate for Lumineers. As I mentioned earlier, in my experience, the majority of patients are candidates to choose Lumineers over traditional veneers. In fact, 90 percent of patients who come into my office for a Lumineers consultation begin the procedure that day. However, this will not always be the case, and you'll want to know as soon as possible if you should be looking at another treatment option.

In our practice, if you decide to proceed with Lumineers, we begin the process by taking a series of pictures—facial and intraoral—to determine which smile type would work best for you. For example, perhaps your teeth are jagged and you would like a "softer" look. In this case, we might recommend rounded Lumineers to provide a more "feminine" smile.

On the other hand, many of our male patients prefer a more "dominant" or "masculine" look.

Once we have picked the type of smile that will work best for you, in some cases (about 20 percent) we may contour your teeth to reshape them to more pleasant proportions. Contouring requires a drill but no shots, and it removes only nonsensitive tooth structure. For example, if your teeth are sharp, we may round them off. In general, the more pleasant the teeth look before the procedure, the better they will look when the Lumineers

are placed. Even if the Lumineers are taken off, the patient's smile will be enhanced as a result of the contouring. In fact, many patients come in for this procedure alone. In our practice, we include contouring for free with every set of Lumineers. Many patients are concerned about the idea of removing any tooth structure; however, remember that every day of your life you are contouring your teeth when you chew your food. In fact, all of us have longer teeth in our youth than we do when we get older because of natural contouring.

Next, we take a mold of the upper and lower teeth. The patient bites down on a tray filled with putty to create an exact working model of the teeth. This enables the Lumineers laboratory to prepare laminates that will precisely fit the teeth. The mold is then sent off to the laboratory. Also in the first visit, we show the patient a variety of

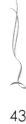
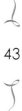

43

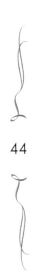

styles and then select the shape and shade of the teeth. This is a highly collaborative process that involves both the artistry of the cosmetic dentist and the personal preference of the patient.

### A Perfect Smile in Only Two Visits!

| Visit One | Visit Two |
|---|---|
| • Consultation | • "Try-on" session |
| • Imaging | • Etching |
| • Contouring | • Bonding |
| • Molding | • Hardening |
| • Shade and shape selection | • Shaping |

After this first appointment is finished, which takes about half an hour, the Lumineers take about two weeks to come back from the laboratory. In the interim, no temporary veneers are needed, as no vital tooth structure has been removed. Once the Lumineers return from the factory, the patient comes in for the second appointment, which takes about an hour and a half. This is the point in which the teeth are prepared and the Lumineers are cemented on.

Before the Lumineers are permanently affixed, we give the patient a chance to see what they will look like by applying "try-it" paste to the Lumineers and fixing them to the teeth temporarily. After the patient approves of his or her new smile, the dentist must *condition* the Lumineers to ensure that they adhere to the bonding agent. This involves lightly etching the interior of the Lumineers with hydrofluoric acid to create more surface area for the bond to adhere to. We then etch the surface of the teeth with phosphoric acid to ensure bonding. Next, we apply a bonding agent (a resin cement) to the Lumineers as well as to the teeth.

44

## *Lumineers versus Traditional Veneers*

| Traditional veneers | Lumineers |
| --- | --- |
| One-year warranty | Ten-year warranty offered by Cerinate |
| Removal of sensitive tooth structure | No removal of sensitive tooth structure |
| Anesthetic shots required | No shots or anesthetic required in most cases |
| Irreversible; cannot be removed due to the grinding down of tooth structure | Reversible; no significant tooth structure removed |
| Temporary veneers required while permanent veneers are being crafted, since sensitive tooth structure will be exposed | No temporary veneers required |

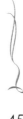

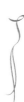

We then affix all the Lumineers to the teeth and harden the resin with a harmless UV curing light, which requires only a few seconds per tooth. Finally, the cosmetic dentist will remove excess cement with a drill and hand instruments (for cosmetic reasons and so the bite comes down correctly). He will then polish the teeth and photograph the results. The patient is then ready to leave with his or her brand-new, natural looking smile.

## *Follow-Up Care*

Now that you have your beautiful new smile, you will want to care for it so it will last you for many years. Fortunately, no special care is required after you get your Lumineers. Treat them as you would your normal teeth, getting periodic cleaning and checkups every six months, as per American Dental Association (ADA) standards. For more information on caring for your cosmetic dentistry, see chapter 7.

### Frequently Asked Questions

The following FAQ list has been reprinted from my website (www.drzaibak.com) and from the Lumineers website:

### How long have Lumineers been around?

Lumineers have been improving smiles for over twenty years. In fact, more than thirteen thousand dentists nationwide use Lumineers and over two hundred fifty thousand people already have Lumineers ... of course, you'd never know because they look so perfect and natural.

### How are Lumineers by Cerinate different from traditional veneer procedures?

Lumineers by Cerinate are unique in that they are contact lens–thin (approximately 0.2 mm) and super translucent. Traditional veneers are fused or bonded to teeth, and generally your dentist will need to grind down the tooth for a good fit. Since Lumineers are so thin, little to no tooth reduction is necessary. In addition, Lumineers resist microleakage and microcracking.

### Do companies other than Cerinate make Lumineers?

*No.* While other companies do produce no-prep veneers, none of these are Lumineers, which are made from proprietary porcelain.

Cerinate was the first company in the market to produce no-prep veneers, and they have had a strong reputation in the industry for more than twenty years. While other companies produce porcelain coverings that are less expensive than Lumineers, only Lumineers offers a ten-year warranty, and in my experience they are the best-looking porcelain coverings on the market.

### How long does the procedure take?

The Lumineers process takes only two visits to your dentist, and the placement of Lumineers on the second visit takes, on average, only about one hour.

### What's involved with a Lumineers procedure?

On the first visit, your dentist will create a precise mold. Then you and your dentist will determine the shade of white that is right for you. After your first visit, your dentist will send

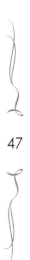

47

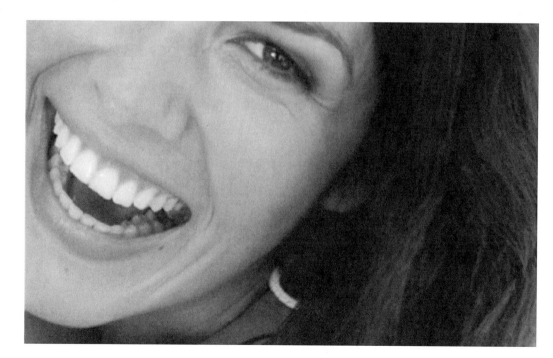

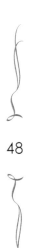 

the mold off to Lumineers Smile Design Studio for your custom Lumineers to be created. With Lumineers, you don't have to wear temporaries. When your dentist receives your custom Lumineers, they are checked for fit and shade. Then during your second visit, your Lumineers are painlessly applied without shots or drilling of sensitive tooth structure. And you're ready to start smiling!

### I've heard that a veneer procedure hurts? Is that true with Lumineers?

It's true that because most traditional veneer procedures require the dentist to remove a substantial amount of tooth structure, there is pain and discomfort involved. Lumineers are completely different, because there is no need for grinding, cutting, or filing of teeth in almost all cases. Consequently, no anesthetic or numbing shots are needed. Plus, no uncomfortable temporaries are re-

quired while you wait for your Lumineers to be created. Once the procedure is completed, there is no postplacement discomfort or sensitivity, which means they will look natural and feel comfortable from the start.

### I think I need braces, but I really don't want to go through the inconvenient, unsightly, and time-intensive process. Can I get Lumineers instead?

In most cases, yes. Your dentist will be able to evaluate your teeth and decide whether orthodontics are necessary. As long as you do not have a severe problem, Lumineers alone will change the shape and alignment of teeth, making them look straighter and more uniform.

### How much does a Lumineers smile cost?

Lumineers by Cerinate are porcelain veneers that the Cerinate Smile Design Studio provides to dentists. Fees are determined by your dentist as he evaluates your smile needs. Lumineer veneer procedures can vary considerably; sometimes only a few Lumineers will dramatically improve your smile and other times more Lumineers are required. Check with your dentist regarding your personal requirements and available payment programs.

### How long will Lumineers last?

Lumineers have unparalleled longevity. Clinical testing has proven that a Lumineers procedure lasts up to twenty years, looking great the whole time. Lumineers by Cerinate also offers a ten-year warranty, which will cover replacing your Lumineers at no

charge if they break. Ask your dentist for details, as certain restrictions do apply.

### Can Lumineers be taken off if I want them removed?

Yes, Lumineers are completely reversible. This is largely because there is no reduction in sensitive tooth structure, so your natural teeth remain intact and strong.

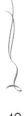

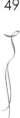

49

### With Lumineers, do I need to use special toothpaste, or should I floss a different way?

Cerinate porcelain is similar in structure to real tooth enamel. Consequently, you should always try to choose a low-abrasion toothpaste that will remove plaque, stains, and tartar gently but effectively.

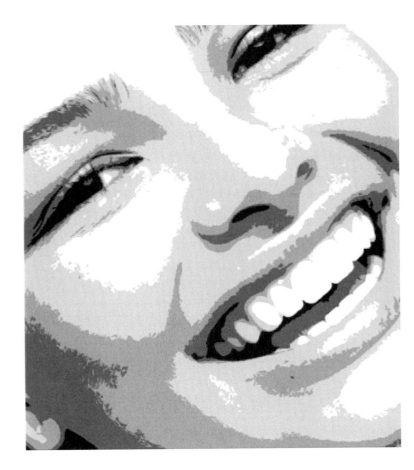

50

## With Lumineers, can I still chew gum and eat my favorite sticky foods, like corn or candy?

There are no limitations to what you can eat or drink, as Lumineers are placed over original teeth in the most durable way possible. However, you should continue to visit your dentist every six months for a checkup and cleaning to keep your Lumineers in good condition and to stay qualified for the warranty.

## Can Lumineers be whitened?

Lumineers, like traditional veneers, cannot be whitened. For this reason, it is important to consult with your dentist about whitening and tooth shade before undergoing this procedure.

### How old should I be to get Lumineers?

To answer that, I'll ask, "How old should you be to have the smile you've always wanted?" There is no reason why teenagers, who are particularly sensitive to cosmetic aesthetics, should have to suffer with crooked, stained, or broken teeth. We do, however, recommend that all permanent teeth have come in before applying Lumineers.

### I have spaces between my teeth. Will Lumineers make my teeth look big and blocky?

Not unless you have very large teeth to begin with. When remodeling your smile, we will make your teeth longer as well as wider.

This will give the smile a better sense of proportion and balance. A balanced, proportioned smile does not look fake; all people see is a great smile, which includes not only the teeth but also the lips, eyes, and cheeks. When you are confident in your smile, it radiates from within.

### I have sensitive teeth. Are Lumineers right for me?

If you have sensitive teeth, your roots may be exposed at the gum line. In this case, Lumineers may actually improve your situation by covering the exposed root. Consult your dentist to see if this is the case for you.

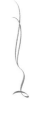

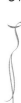

51

# CHAPTER 3

## INVISALIGN—ALIGNING YOUR TEETH FOR BEAUTY AND FUNCTION

There are many reasons to ensure you have straight teeth. Our truest nature is to be aligned and balanced, and we gravitate toward others who exhibit balance in their own bodies—particularly their smile. Depending on the severity of deviation, we tend to judge people who have crooked teeth. Unconsciously, we think of them as less educated, less intelligent, and less mindful of their personal hygiene. In short, we unfairly assume that they are in a poor state of health. Subconsciously, they understand that people think this way, and as a result they smile less, or smile unnaturally. This leads people to believe that they are unhappy, or worse, that they do not like us.

Even aside from one's appearance, there are legitimate health concerns that come with having crooked teeth. Teeth out of alignment may wear faster than normal, they are more prone to cavities, and they increase the likelihood of various ailments, such as TMJ dysfunction, which is discussed later in this chapter.

Traditionally, crooked teeth have been treated with dental braces, which use metal brackets, wires, and rubber bands to apply constant pressure to the teeth, causing them to move over time. While there is no doubt that traditional braces get the job done, they have many drawbacks: They are visually unappealing, particularly on adults. They are impossible to remove temporarily, making it more difficult to clean your teeth—increasing the chance of cavities—and increasing the chance of sports injury. They also require you to sacrifice certain types of

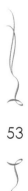

food, which can break the delicate mechanisms that hold everything in place.

Thankfully, today there are many options when it comes to teeth alignment, making it a more attractive option for adults. For example, there are now "clear" braces, which use ceramic brackets instead of traditional metal brackets and clear ties instead of metal wires. This makes them indistinguishable from the teeth. There are also lingual braces, which fit to the back of the teeth, making them invisible to anyone standing in front of you. However, in these cases you still have to be careful about what comes near your braces, and there is nearly continuous discomfort due to the constant pressure being applied.

This is why *Invisalign*, in my opinion, is the best option for teeth straightening today. Invisalign is a clear, removable plastic mouthpiece that's placed over your teeth. Since these are clear plastic aligners, they are virtually undetectable. Unlike braces, they can be removed at will, meaning you can take them out when you eat, clean your teeth, and play sports.

As you might expect, Invisalign is very popular among teenagers who want straight teeth but don't like the idea of a mouth full of metal. In my experience, parents of teens love Invisalign—and not only for cosmetic reasons. There are practical reasons as well. One is sports. Teens with traditional braces who play sports with any contact (including soccer) are at high risk of injury if they are hit in the mouth. With Invisalign, they don't need to worry about such injuries, and if additional mouth protection is required (e.g., a mouth guard for football or hockey), all they need to do is remove the mouthpiece during the game. Despite our best efforts as parents, teens are also notoriously prone to damaging their braces by eating the wrong foods. With Invisalign, this is not a concern, since the mouthpiece is removed during mealtimes. Teens are free to eat as they would normally. They simply need to clean their teeth following meals before they reinsert the mouthpiece—a practice we should all be doing anyway! In this way, Invisalign actually promotes good dental hygiene among teens.

In the following picture, you see another result that can occur with the use of braces. This patient came to our office after having received metal braces from another dentist. Limited in her ability to floss and brush, this fifteen-year-old girl ended up developing a form of gingivitis, which you can see in the swollen and excess gum tissue around her upper teeth.

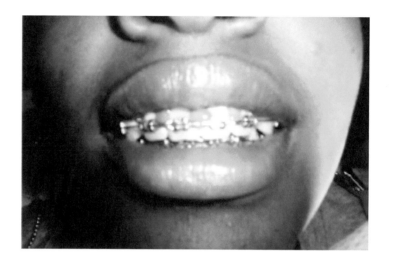

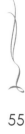

55

## Who Is Eligible for Invisalign?

For its many benefits, I always recommend Invisalign to patients if they are eligible candidates. Thanks to advancements in Invisalign technology, it can handle most alignment problems traditionally corrected with braces. Invisalign is used to treat the following conditions:

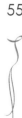

- Spaced teeth
- Overly crowded teeth
- Crossbite (upper and lower jaw misaligned)
- Underbite
- Overbite

56

In rare circumstances—for instance, if teeth are extremely crooked or crowded or if there is severe malocclusion (misaligned bite)—a patient may not be a candidate for Invisalign. In such cases, the patient may require oral surgery (including jaw fracturing) to correct their bite. *Patients cannot determine on their own if their bite is too severe, as severity is defined differently in different people.* Therefore, patients shouldn't rule themselves out based on what they have read. The only way to know what treatment is suitable for you is to visit an Invisalign certified dentist.

> *Only an Invisalign certified dentist can determine if you are a candidate for Invisalign.*

### The Invisalign Procedure

The first thing you need to do if you are considering Invisalign is locate an experienced Invisalign preferred provider in your area to book your consultation. As with Lumineers, we recommend expanding your search to include nearby cities, but keep in mind that you will need periodic readjustments, so you will need to go to this dentist more than once. We recommend visiting a few providers to find a doctor with whom you are comfortable. You will want to ensure that this doctor is certified with Invisalign and has received the proper training.

During the consultation, your dentist will decide if you are a candidate for Invisalign. Please resist the temptation to perform this assessment yourself. Thanks to modern advances in Invisalign technology, more people than ever are candidates for the process. Although Invisalign does offer a self-assessment form on their website, only an Invisalign certified dentist can truly determine whether you are a candidate. During the consultation, you can also ask about the cost of treatment, including whether your insurance will cover any of the fees.

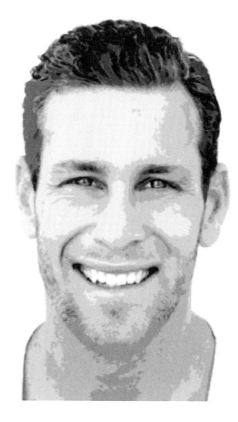

outside of your mouth (eight pictures in total), and then send them to Invisalign by e-mail. Invisalign will use this information to create a 3-D model of your mouth. The image is sent to your dentist, who will use this model to create an individual treatment plan based on your specific needs. He will also be able to show you what your mouth will look like after the treatment is complete. Once the patient sees the model and the proposed plan, he or she will have the chance to *approve* it before treatment begins. This is done in close consultation with the dentist.

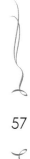

To begin the process, the dentist will take X-rays, intraoral pictures, and pictures of the

Next, a series of custom-made clear aligners will be fabricated specifically for you.

58

This takes approximately three weeks. Unlike traditional braces, these aligners are made of a smooth plastic, which will not irritate the inside of your mouth. Once the aligners have been delivered to the dentist, the patient comes in for a fitting to ensure that the aligners are working properly. Often it will be necessary to place attachments on the mouthpiece, which attach the teeth to the aligner more securely, helping the teeth move faster. This is strictly optional as part of the treatment plan. From this point onward, all you need to do is consistently wear the aligners, removing them only when you eat, brush or floss your teeth, or participate in a contact sport. Approximately *every two weeks*, you will receive a new set of aligners, which will advance you to the next stage of your treatment. It is also recommended you check in with your dentist *every six weeks* to see what kind of progress you are making. You may experience some mild discomfort following adjustments, but this will diminish after a day or two and can be treated with a mild painkiller, such as ibuprofen. In some cases, the dentist will evaluate the progress part way through the treatment and determine that a *refinement* is needed. This involves changing the shape of the aligner to correct any issues that have come up (e.g., a problem with your bite). *Be sure to ask your dentist how many refinements are included with your treatment plan.* (In my office, all refinements are included with the treatment plan.) The length of time it will take to complete the Invisalign process will vary from patient to patient; talk to your dentist about your timeline. At the end of the treatment, you may need to wear a retainer to ensure the teeth do not shift back to their previous position. The same would be required with traditional braces.

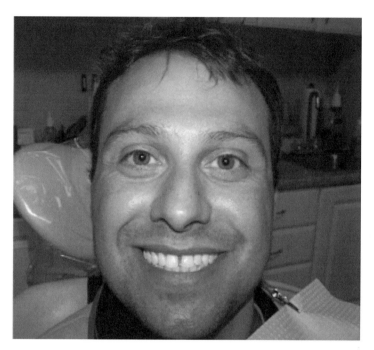

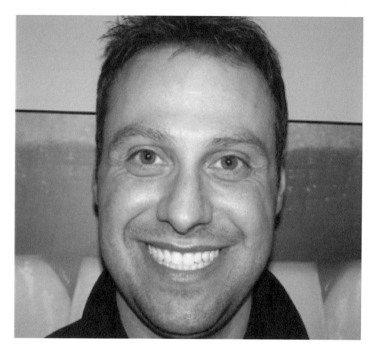

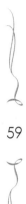

Mario was a fun-loving guy when he came in to see us. The gap between his teeth never stopped him from smiling, but it did make him self-conscious at times.

Mario underwent Invisalign treatment for nine months to correct the bite, as well as cosmetic contouring. Closing the gap made him more confident in his smile.

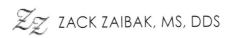 

### *Braces versus Invisalign*

| Traditional Braces | Invisalign |
| --- | --- |
| Extra care required when brushing teeth to ensure wires do not break | Brush your teeth as you normally would, as aligners are removable; rinse out aligners separately, using lukewarm water or Invisalign cleaning kit |
| Extra care required when eating; hard and/or chewy foods not recommended | Eat as you would normally, as aligners are removed when you're eating |
| Extra care required when playing sports, to ensure braces are not damaged | Play as you normally would, since aligners can be removed |

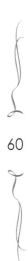

60

### *Getting the Most out of Your Invisalign Aligners*

Invisalign offers many advantages over traditional braces—they are more comfortable, better looking, and easier to care for. However, they do require some vigilance on the part of the patient. For the treatment to be effective, the patient must wear the mouthpiece at least twenty hours a day, removing them only when necessary. It is important to remove them when eating or drinking anything other than water to prevent staining. Teeth should be brushed after every meal, the patient should floss every day, and the mouthpiece should be rinsed regularly to ensure no food particles or sugars are trapped between the mouthpiece and the teeth. On the upside, this continued vigilance makes us more aware of our dental health, which is an area where most of us could stand to improve.

In my experience, the biggest problem is that patients tend to lose their aligners. This often happens when they are out at a party or some other event and take them out while they're eating. If this happens, it is important to contact your dentist immediately so he can order a new set of aligners. The cost to replace a lost aligner is roughly one hundred dollars.

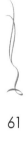

### Brian, thirty-six

After college, I got married and got a job as an engineer. My career was going well, but unfortunately my marriage didn't work out, and twelve years after college I found myself back on the dating market at the age of thirty-four.

My life was going well, and I should have been confident, but I never felt truly comfortable with my appearance, and I felt that this was the only thing holding me back when meeting women. I'd had braces as a child for a number of years, but afterward I never wore my retainer, despite the constant nagging of my orthodontist. Turns out she was right. As I got older, my teeth started moving back to their original position.

I knew I wanted to do something about it, but I remembered the pain and awkwardness that I felt as a teenager wearing braces. I had been recently promoted to a managerial position, and I couldn't imagine showing up one day with a mouthful of metal (particularly in construction, which can be a tough crowd).

I asked Dr. Zaibak about what I should do, and he told me about Invisalign. I'd never heard of it, but he assured me that it had been around for a while and that many of his patients had gotten great results. I thought I had to go to an orthodontist to get that kind of treatment—really, that's the only reason I went to him that day, to get a referral—but he told me that he could do it right in his office. I was surprised and relieved. Dr. Zaibak had always taken such good care of me, doing all my cleanings for years and whitening my teeth a couple of years ago.

The treatment itself was faster than I thought, and barely anyone noticed. After a while it became completely natural to wear my mouthpiece. It was like putting on my glasses. I just forgot it was there. When I was done, no one asked me if I had gotten my teeth fixed—I suppose no one really paid that much attention to the way my teeth looked before—but my female friends often told me that I looked happier these days. And I *was* happier. It was like I had put off some important task for a long time, which never really allowed me to relax even when I wasn't thinking about it. Now that I had done it, I felt a great sense of relief.

As I said, I had been recently promoted, and I had planned to make this my treat to myself, and so I earmarked my bonus that year for the treatment. However, I was pleasantly surprised to learn that my company insurance plan would pick up more than half the cost of the treatment! I put the money I got back from insurance into a Caribbean vacation with my new girlfriend. Those were without a doubt the best vacation snaps I have ever taken!

## Frequently Asked Questions about Invisalign

The following information can be found on Invisalign's website:

### What are aligners made of, and what do they look like?

The virtually invisible aligners, which are made of a thermoplastic material uniquely developed for the Invisalign treatment plan, look similar to teeth-whitening trays. A series of Invisalign aligners are custom-made for you, to move your teeth in the sequence determined by your doctor.

### How do the aligners straighten teeth?

Over the course of treatment, you will be supplied with a series of aligners. Each aligner will make slight adjustments to tooth position, a process that is mapped out in advance by your doctor, specifically for your situation. When the aligners are placed on the teeth, they cause the teeth to gradually shift from their current position. After approximately two weeks, you will begin using the next set of aligners, which will continue the teeth straightening process.

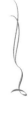

### How will Invisalign effectively move my teeth?

Through the use of our patented thermoplastic design, Invisalign aligners move your teeth through the appropriate placement of controlled force. The main difference is that Invisalign not only controls the force, but also the timing of the force application. During each stage, only certain teeth are allowed to move. These movements are determined by your doctor as he or she maps out your unique Invisalign treatment plan.

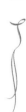

63

### What are the primary benefits of Invisalign?

Invisalign aligners are virtually invisible. No one may even notice that you're wearing them, making Invisalign a seamless fit with your lifestyle. Invisalign aligners are removable. For the best results and a timely outcome, aligners should be worn for twenty to twenty-two hours per day. However, unlike with braces, you have the flexibility to remove your aligners to eat and drink what you want during treatment. And you can also remove the aligners to brush and floss as you normally would, for fresh breath and good oral hygiene. There are no metal brackets or wires that could cause irritation to your mouth, an advantage over traditional braces. Plus, since your office visits during treatment don't involve metal or wire adjustments, you'll likely spend less time in the doctor's chair. Invisalign allows you to view your virtual results and treatment plan before you start so you can see how your straight teeth will look when your treatment is complete. Instead of imagining how much better it can be, you'll be able to see it for yourself.

### Will Invisalign treatment be painful?

While Invisalign moves your teeth without the pain and anxiety metal braces can cause, some people experience temporary discomfort for a few days at the beginning of each new stage of treatment. This is normal and is typically described as a feeling of pressure. It's also a sign that Invisalign is working, as it moves your teeth to their final destination. This discomfort typically goes away in a couple of days.

### Will wearing Invisalign aligners affect my speech?

Similar to other orthodontic treatments, Invisalign aligners may temporarily affect the speech of some people, and you may have a slight lisp for a day or two. However, as your tongue gets used to having aligners in your mouth, any lisp caused by the aligners should disappear.

### What's the best way to clean my aligners?

The best way to clean your aligners is to use the Invisalign cleaning kit, available for order at www.invisalignstore.com. As a secondary method, however, your aligners can also be cleaned by brushing them and rinsing them in lukewarm water.

### What happens after treatment to prevent my teeth from moving again?

This varies from person to person and depends on the outcome of the treatment. Some patients might need a positioner, or conventional retainer. Other patients might need a clear plastic retainer similar to the ones Invisalign makes, such as Align Technology's Vivera Retainer, which is worn at night. Discuss this with your dentist. Every patient is different, and outcomes vary.

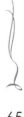

65

### TMJ Dysfunction

As I mentioned earlier, we often mistakenly assume that people with crooked teeth are in a poor state of health. In fact, this often turns out to be the case. Teeth alignment isn't just about cosmetics. Having a misaligned bite can profoundly affect your quality of life. This is particularly true among patients who suffer

from TMJ dysfunction. *Temporomandibular joint (TMJ) dysfunction* refers to inflammation of the temporomandibular joint, which connects the mandible to the skull. Its symptoms include the following:

- Chronic headache

- Nausea

- Dizziness

- Hearing loss

- Tinnitus (ringing in the ears)

- Jaw, cheek, tooth, or shoulder pain

The American Dental Association estimates that 30 percent of all people in the United States suffer from this syndrome; however, people are often unaware that they have it. All they know is that they are suffering from chronic headaches or pain. They take pain medications to treat the symptoms, but never get to the root cause. If you are experiencing any of the symptoms above, it is important to visit your dentist to determine whether you have TMJ dysfunction. Only your dentist can say for certain whether this is the case.

While the reasons for TMJ dysfunction are various, one of the most common causes is a problem with your bite. Even a single misaligned tooth can cause your jaw to overcompensate, causing strain and discomfort. Or you may have one or more unhealthy teeth, causing you to chew primarily on one side so you don't put pressure on them. As a result, you put more pressure on your temporomandibular joint, which can lead to TMJ dysfunction and the degeneration of that joint. This in turn may affect other parts of your musculoskeletal system. As we stress often in this book, all the areas of our body make up a highly interconnected system.

Therefore, when we apply force with our mouths, it's important that the force is distributed evenly over the entire area of the mouth to keep everything in equilibrium.

## Treatment Options

There are several ways to align the teeth, enhancing the appearance of your smile and the functionality of your bite. Below, we will look at the various options.

**Invisalign:** I once saw a new patient in his thirties who had been having daily headaches for almost ten years. Ten years! He'd seen many doctors, but all they could do was offer him pain meds. He eventually came to believe nothing could be done and he would have to live with his pain. When I saw him, his teeth were actually quite healthy and mostly aligned. However, I could tell his bite was a little off in the rear. I told him that

if he wore braces, his headaches might go away. He gave me a puzzled look. None of the many doctors he had seen had even brought up this possibility. Besides, he told me, he was a professional in his thirties and braces were for teenagers. He thought he would look silly wearing them.

I responded, "Would you mind looking silly for a short period if it meant living without pain for the rest of your life? And besides," I added, "with Invisalign, they'll be practically undetectable."

He began the treatment, and within a month, to his amazement, he woke up one morning with no headache. No headache all that day and night. Within a relatively short time, all his headaches disappeared. Suffice it to say, he was very grateful.

**Contouring:** In addition to being a cosmetic procedure, contouring can also improve

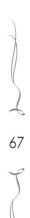

67

68

the function of the teeth. After evaluating the bite, if the dentist detects premature contact between the teeth (if some teeth are making contact before the rest), he or she can contour the teeth to create a more harmonious bite. This process involves using a drill or laser to remove a small portion of the surface enamel to reshape the tooth. The process is not highly invasive and does not require anesthetic. In fact, your teeth undergo contouring every day, each time you bite down. This is why the same person's teeth at fifty will be shorter than they were at twenty.

**Bite splints:** If you have TMJ dysfunction and contouring is not a solution, bite splints (also known as night guards) may be an option. A bite splint is a small "cushion" that fits over the teeth, ensuring there isn't any excessive pressure when biting. This also takes pressure off the temporomandibular joint. To prepare the splints, the dentist first takes a mold of the teeth. He then sends it to the lab, which produces the mouthpiece for the patient. Bite splints have the advantages of being easy to make, easy to use, and inexpensive. However, their overall effectiveness is a continuing matter of debate in the dental community.

**Braces:** In more severe cases, where neither contouring nor splints are likely to improve the bite, a more invasive realigning of the jaw may be required. In these cases, braces may be required. Braces align the teeth by applying force over time. All braces consist of the following basic parts:

- Brackets (made of metal or ceramic, these are affixed to the teeth)
- Bonding material (the material used to affix brackets to the teeth)

- Arch wire (these are attached to the brackets, applying force to the teeth)
- Elastics (these apply additional force to the brackets)

Braces move the teeth when pressure is applied to the brackets in a particular direction determined by the orthodontist over a specified duration of time. In addition, headgear is occasionally needed to keep the teeth aligned, and elastics are used to exert additional force on the brackets. Pressure must be exerted very slowly to prevent the pa-

tient from losing their teeth, as the periodontal membrane is stretched and compressed during this process. This is why it takes more than two years, on average, to realign the teeth using braces.

**Botox:** Although not commonly known, another way to treat certain types of TMJ dysfunction is with Botox. It works by relaxing the muscles (the masseter and temporalis) that pull on the jaw and the joint, thus decreasing the clenching and stress placed on the temporomandibular joint. This can bring relief from the symptoms of TMJ dysfunction.

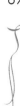

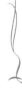

69

# CHAPTER 4

## ZOOM 2 WHITENING—
## THE WHITEST SMILE YOU'VE EVER HAD

Part of having a great smile is having a *bright* smile. As we get older, our teeth tend to darken, losing their whiteness and luster. When this happens, we may be more reluctant to show them when we smile, and this can give the people we meet a poor first impression. This may also affect the way we smile in photographs, making us self-conscious and camera shy or causing us to contort our mouth into an unnatural-looking close-lipped smile. Perhaps we even come to avoid cameras altogether. Thankfully, there are ways to restore the brightness of your smile. We have already discussed Lumineers as a way to do this. While Lumineers or even traditional veneers offer the option

of a dazzling Hollywood smile, not everyone is a candidate for one of these processes, be it for financial or other reasons. However, thanks to significant advances in whitening methods, just about everyone can have a brighter smile. While none of these methods are permanent (as they are with Lumineers or traditional veneers), their duration has improved dramatically, and so has their ease of use. In this chapter, we will discuss some of the various whitening options, focusing primarily on Zoom 2, the most advanced whitening product offered to date.

### *Why Do Teeth Get Dark?*

First off, we would like to make it clear that there is no such thing as a "normal" tooth color. Much as people have varying skin tones and hair colors, everyone has their own baseline tooth color which is the maximum

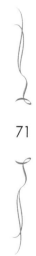

brightness they could achieve. Between professional cleanings, they will likely pick up surface stains, left by foods and other products, such as coffee and tea, cola, red wine, pasta sauce, berries, and tobacco. Teeth also naturally darken as we age as a result of changes in the mineral structure and enamel. They may also permanently darken due to injury or certain medications, such as tetracycline. In cases of permanent darkening,

the patient would not be eligible for whitening and would need to apply Lumineers to brighten their smile. However, in most cases that involve simple yellowing of the teeth, whitening will dramatically improve the appearance of your smile, making your teeth up to ten shades whiter.

## Types of Whitening

Several different types of whitening systems are available. The most popular professional whitening systems are in-office bleaching and at-home bleaching. There are also non-dental systems available (at shopping malls, spas, etc.), but we do not recommend these, for reasons we will discuss. In addition, there are various products marketed as "whitening," including toothpastes, mouthwashes, and chewing gums. We will discuss these various methods as well.

72

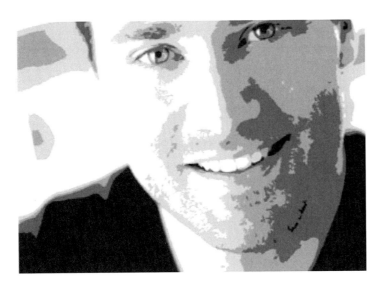

**Zoom 2 (in-office laser bleaching):** This professional system, available in the dental office, offers dramatic results. It involves putting bleach on your teeth for just one hour, resulting in much whiter teeth. This is the method I recommend to patients who have an event to attend within a week's time (such as a wedding or a photography session) and want whiter teeth.

Like any cosmetic dentistry procedure, the process begins with an initial consultation with your dentist. The first thing the dentist will do is determine your eligibility for whitening. If you have discoloration due to tetracycline staining or injury, you are not a candidate for Zoom 2 (or any of the whitening systems described here). In this consultation, the dentist will also examine your mouth, including your teeth and gums. If you have any cavities, they will need to be treated before any whitening process can begin, as

the bleaching materials could further erode tooth structure in this case. In addition, if you have extremely sensitive gums or receding gums, you will want to consult with your dentist beforehand.

Once your dentist determines that you are a candidate, you can talk about treatment options, including selecting a shade and discussing the results that you can expect to get. It is important to be realistic with your expectations. (If you have extremely dark teeth, you may not be able to get an extremely bright smile with whitening alone.) At this time, you can also discuss whether you want to undergo the treatment in the office or at home.

In our practice, we always disclose that a small percentage of patients experience some sensitivity during the procedure. Sensitivity occurs when hydrogen peroxide, a

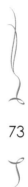

73

74

bleaching agent used in whitening treatments, oozes onto the gums and enters the roots, causing inflammation. If we know the patient is interested in whitening, we advise them to use a sensitivity toothpaste (e.g., Sensodyne) for up to two weeks before the procedure. We also find that fluoride treatments can help reduce sensitivity leading up to the whitening. These are available at most pharmacies, usually in a rinse or gel form. You can also continue to use these treatments following the whitening if sensitivity persists, but the good news is that tooth sensitivity due to bleaching always goes away within a couple of days.

To start the Zoom 2 procedure, we set the patient down in a comfortable massage chair in front of a TV screen, which they can watch during treatment. Alternatively, they can listen to music on a portable media device. Next, we take a couple of protective measures to ensure that the procedure is as safe and comfortable as possible. These include applying a dental dam over the lips and gums to ensure that none of the bleaching solution gets into sensitive areas and providing UV glasses to protect the eyes from the high-intensity light used during the process. Next, we apply the bleaching solution, a gel with a high concentration of hydrogen peroxide. Then we turn on the Zoom 2 lamp, which acts as a catalyst, allowing the hydrogen peroxide to penetrate the enamel. This process takes fifteen minutes and is repeated two or three times, for a total of up to one hour. Following treatment, we give the patient instructions on what not to eat and drink for the next forty-eight hours, and then the patient is free to go home and enjoy their dazzling new smile.

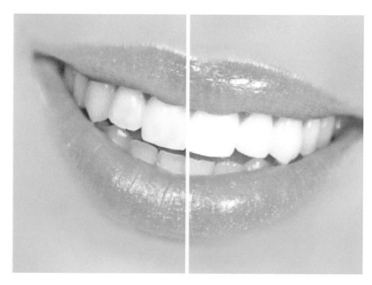

Before and after pictures of teeth whitening.

**Take-home trays:** In take-home systems, the dentist creates a plastic mold fitted to your teeth, which we call a "tray." A solution is put into the tray, which then fits over your teeth. It is activated simply by time (no laser, obviously), so it takes longer—usually about two weeks, with treatments being done most every day. You will get a similar result to the

laser treatment, and the upside is you have the system to use for the rest of your life. All you need is to purchase more of the solution, which you put inside the trays. The disadvantage with take-home systems is that they take longer to achieve the desired results. There are a number of precautions the patient can take to get the most out of take-home systems. I recommend the following:

- *Don't put in too much bleaching gel.* Trays are designed so that you need to put in only a small amount of gel each time. Have your dentist show you how much to put in, and then put in the same amount every time you use the tray. This will ensure the solution does not get under the gum line, which can cause the roots to inflame, resulting in unnecessary sensitivity over a long duration.

- *Don't put bleaching gel on your back teeth, or on the backside of your front*

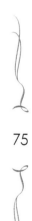

75

*teeth.* Only put gel on parts of your teeth that are visible. Otherwise you will go through your gel very quickly. In most cases, you only need to apply gel to the front of your first eight teeth, top and bottom.

- *Discontinue treatment when you reach your brightest shade.* All of us have our own natural tooth shade. There is no reason to continue bleaching once we have reached that shade. If you have been wearing bleaching trays for three or four days and have seen no significant color change, you have likely attained your brightest natural shade.

- *Get regular dental examinations.* This goes for everyone, but it is especially important if you plan to use whitening trays at home. If cavities develop, these need to be treated before any whitening is done;

otherwise, you risk eroding the enamel even further.

- *Do not use bleaching trays if you are pregnant or nursing.* The chemicals in the bleaching trays will enter the bloodstream, so it is important that pregnant or nursing women do not attempt whitening (at home or in office) during this period.

**Nondental treatments:** You may see teeth whitening offered in commercial settings, such as shopping malls, kiosks, spas, and cruise ships. Clients are often lured in by the affordable prices of these treatments, which are often offered as part of an aesthetics package. In these settings, the clinician applies a high concentration bleaching solution, much as you would at home with take-home trays. We do not recommend these treatments. First, these practitioners are not

76

qualified to assess whether you are a suitable candidate for whitening. They cannot identify intrinsically dark teeth, and they cannot check for cavities or identify other oral issues that might be cause for concern. Second, whereas a dentist is trained to administer these treatments, a clinician might be vastly underexperienced. This may lead to improper application of the bleaching material, which may lead to sensitivity. Third, there are no government bodies regulating these practitioners. Getting your teeth whitened is not like getting your hair done; it is a complicated procedure with many variables, and you are better off getting it done by a trained, certified professional. If you're looking for a more economical whitening solution, you're much better off getting take-home trays from your dentist and having him or her show you how to use them safely.

**Over-the-counter treatments:** These include products like toothpastes, rinses, and strips. Of these products, strips have been known to provide some whitening, but the concentrations of the active ingredient (usually hydrogen peroxide) are usually too low to provide effective whitening. Also, they may cause sensitivity, since they are modeled on a generic mouth profile, meaning that they might not fit the user properly. As for so-called whitening toothpastes, chewing gums, rinses, etc., while they do contain the active ingredient in professional bleaching agents, the concentration is very low, and they do not remain on your teeth long enough to be effective.

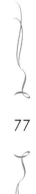

77

## Following Your Whitening Treatment

Within the first forty-eight hours of treatment, we recommend that you do not consume foods and other products that may stain your teeth. These include coffee, tea, cola, berries, red pasta sauce, and red wine. Afterward, it is recommended that you brush your teeth immediately after consuming such foods (which we would advise everyone to do, regardless of whether they have had a whitening treatment). You may also want to avoid consuming hot or cold foods and citric acid (found in orange juice, lemons, etc.) for the first forty-eight hours, in case there is sensitivity.

Immediately following treatment, you may also experience gum burning or gum bleaching (where the gums have turned white). This is a result of the bleaching product coming into contact with your gums. Do not be alarmed, as this discoloration or burning is only temporary and will disappear within a day or two.

---

### Mary, twenty-eight

My teeth had never been truly white. Even in high school they had a yellowish tint. I didn't seem to notice in the past, but I became increasingly self-conscious about it through the years, and by the time I was in college I was consciously avoiding the camera.

When my picture began popping up regularly on social media sites, I really started to notice the way my smile looked. I would always keep my mouth closed when I knew that the camera was on me, but occasionally someone would tag a photo of me when I didn't realize they'd taken my picture. I was horrified at what I saw! Digital photography today is so clear that it picks up everything! I was so embarrassed at the thought of what I looked like that I soon stopped smiling altogether just to make sure I wouldn't be caught on film again.

Other than my smile, I have always thought of myself as quite attractive, and I remember seeing pictures of myself as a child where I would grin from ear to ear, showing off my smile. I looked so genuinely happy then. It made me sad to see those pictures, knowing that I never smile like that today. I've never considered myself an un-happy person, but every time I saw a picture of myself, I saw this tense, unconfident person look-ing back at me.

One day I decided I'd had enough, and I called Doctor Zaibak. He told me about Zoom 2. I had heard of the procedure, but I was a little worried about it, because I heard that it was painful. He told me that I might have some sensitivity but that I could reduce it by brushing with Sensodyne before my treatment. I decided to give it a shot, and I couldn't believe how easy it actually was!

An hour later I was out of the office, and there was virtually no sensitivity at all. I almost started crying when I saw how my smile looked. I would recommend the procedure to anyone who isn't happy with the color of their teeth. My only re-gret is not doing it years sooner!

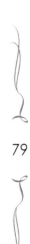

## Frequently Asked Questions about Teeth Whitening

The following FAQ is taken from the Zoom! website.

## What is Zoom! tooth whitening?

Zoom! is a bleaching process that lightens discoloration of enamel and dentin. You may have seen the Zoom! process used on ABC's *Extreme Makeover*.

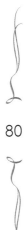

### How long does Zoom! Chairside Whitening take?

The complete procedure takes less than an hour. The procedure begins with a preparation period followed by as little as forty-five minutes of bleaching. (A cleaning is recommended prior to the actual Zoom! whitening session.)

### How does the Zoom! in-office system work?

The Zoom! light-activated whitening gel's active ingredient is hydrogen peroxide. As the hydrogen peroxide is broken down, oxygen enters the enamel and dentin, bleaching colored substances while the structure of the tooth is unchanged. The Zoom! light aids in activating the hydrogen peroxide and helps it penetrate the surface of the tooth. A study has shown that use of the Zoom! lamp increases the effectiveness of the Zoom! gel by 26 percent or more, giving an average improvement of up to eight shades.

### What will I experience during the Zoom! in-office procedure?

During the procedure, patients may comfortably watch television or listen to music. Individuals with a strong gag reflex or anxiety may have difficulty undergoing the entire procedure.

### How long do the results last?

By following some simple postwhitening care instructions, your teeth will always be lighter than they were before. To keep your teeth looking their best, we recommend flossing, brushing twice daily, and occasional touch-ups with Zoom! Weekender or Nite White gel.

These are professional formula products designed specifically to keep your teeth their brightest. They are available only through your dental professional.

## Are there any side effects?

Sensitivity during the treatment may occur with some patients. The Zoom! light generates minimal heat, which is the usual source of discomfort. On rare occasions, minor tingling sensations are experienced immediately after the procedure, but always dissipate. You can also ask your dentist to supply you with anti-sensitivity toothpaste for use prior to treatment.

## What causes tooth discoloration?

There are many causes. The most common include aging and consumption of staining substances, such as coffee, tea, colas, tobacco, red wine, etc. During tooth formation, consumption of tetracycline, certain other antibiotics, or excessive fluoride may also cause tooth discoloration.

## Do many people whiten their teeth?

More people than you might imagine. A bright, sparkling smile can make a big difference for everyone. The Zoom! Chairside Whitening System makes it easier and faster than ever before.

## Who may benefit from tooth whitening?

Almost anyone. However, treatment may not be as effective for some as it is for others. Your dental professional can determine if you are a viable candidate for this procedure through a thorough oral exam, including a shade assessment.

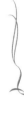

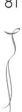

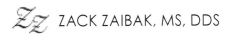 

### *Is whitening safe?*

Yes. Extensive research and clinical studies indicate that whitening teeth under the supervision of a dentist is safe. In fact, many dentists consider whitening the safest cosmetic dental procedure available. As with any tooth whitening product, Zoom! is not recommended for children under thirteen years of age and pregnant or lactating women.

# CHAPTER 5

## BRIDGES, CROWNS, BONDING, SNAP-ON SMILES, AND GUM LIFTS

In this chapter, we will talk about some other cosmetic procedures not discussed previously.

### Porcelain Crowns (Caps)

A crown (or cap) is a covering that encases the entire tooth surface, restoring it to its original shape and size. A crown protects and strengthens tooth structure that cannot be restored with fillings or other types of restorations.

Although there are several types of crowns, porcelain crowns are the most popular, because they resemble your natural teeth.

They are highly durable and last many years, but like most dental restorations, they may eventually need to be replaced. Porcelain crowns are made to match the shape, size, and color or your teeth, giving you a natural, long-lasting, beautiful smile.

### Reasons for Crowns

- Broken or fractured teeth
- Cosmetic enhancement
- Decayed teeth
- Fractured fillings
- Large fillings
- Root canal

### Procedure

A crown procedure usually requires two appointments. During the first appointment, the

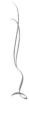

dentist takes several highly accurate molds (or impressions) that will be used to create your custom crown. A mold will also be used to create a temporary crown, which will stay on your tooth for approximately two weeks, while your new crown is fabricated by a dental laboratory.

While the tooth is numb, the dentist will prepare the tooth by removing any decay and shaping the surface to properly fit the crown. Once this happens, your temporary crown will be placed with temporary cement and your bite will be checked to ensure you are biting properly.

At your second appointment, your temporary crown will be removed, the tooth will be cleaned, and your new crown will be carefully placed to ensure the spacing and bite are accurate.

You will be given care instructions and encouraged to have regular dental visits to check your new crown.

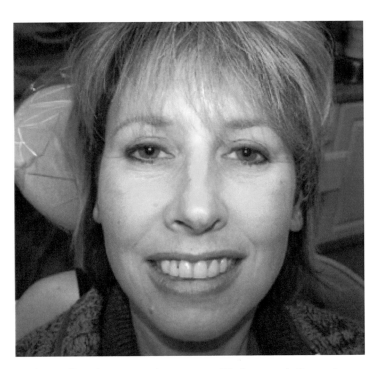

This patient was unhappy with her existing dental work and wanted a total smile makeover.

84

## Bonding

Bonding involves the direct application of tooth-colored composite resin and is typically used to create a more attractive smile.

Bonding can be employed to change the size or shape of your teeth, creating a smile that appears more symmetrical and free of spaces. This single-visit procedure provides a fast solution for a more attractive smile and may eliminate the need for orthodontic treatment.

Tooth stains and discoloration that resist professional teeth whitening procedures may also be masked by bonding. Although bonding may not be as long lasting as veneers or crowns, it is definitely a more economical way to achieve an attractive smile.

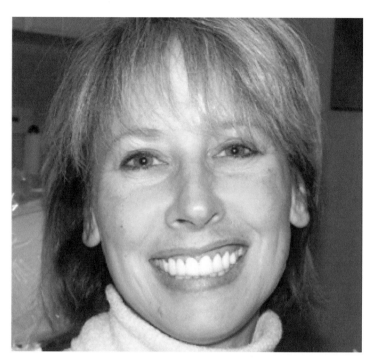

We did a full-mouth reconstruction, replacing the old crowns and bridges with high-end ceramics, such as Lava crowns and daVinci veneers. We also did gum contouring and whitened her teeth. When she saw the end result, her face lit up with an enormous smile.

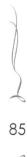

85

## Dental Bridges

A dental bridge is a fixed (nonremovable) appliance, which provides an excellent way to replace missing teeth.

There are several types of bridges. The "traditional bridge" is the most popular and is usually made of porcelain fused to metal. Porcelain fixed bridges are most popular because they most closely resemble your natural teeth. This type of bridge consists of two crowns that go over two anchoring teeth (or abutment teeth), and are attached to pontics (artificial teeth) that fill the gap created by one or more missing teeth.

Dental bridges are highly durable and will last many years. However, they may need replacement, or need to be recemented due to normal wear.

## Reasons for a Fixed Bridge

- Fill space of missing teeth
- Maintain facial shape
- Prevent remaining teeth from drifting out of position
- Restore chewing and speaking ability
- Restore a smile
- Upgrade from a removable partial denture to a permanent dental appliance

## Procedure

Getting a bridge usually requires two or more visits. While your teeth are numb, the two anchoring teeth are prepared by removing a portion of enamel to allow for a crown. Next, a highly accurate impression (mold) is made, which is then sent to a dental laboratory where the bridge will be fabricated. In addition, the dentist will give you a temporary bridge that you can wear for several weeks until your next appointment.

At the second visit, your permanent bridge will be carefully checked, adjusted, and cemented to achieve a proper fit. Occasionally your dentist will only temporarily cement the bridge, allowing your teeth and tissue time to get used to the new bridge. The new bridge will be permanently cemented at a later time.

You will receive care instructions at the conclusion of your treatment. Proper brushing, flossing, and regular dental visits will aid in the life of your new permanent bridge.

## Snap-On Smiles

A Snap-On Smile is an excellent alternative for people who desire a smile makeover but cannot afford Lumineers. A Snap-On Smile is a thin, strong covering made of a high-tech proprietary resin. It is designed to fit over your teeth, covering any stains, chips, gaps, or missing teeth. It is available for both upper and lower teeth. No drilling is involved, and no shots. You can eat and drink with it, although it is not recommended that you chew gum while wearing it.

### Reasons for a Snap-On Smile

- Gaps, crooked, stained, or missing teeth
- Removal of a partial denture
- Ineligible for bridges or implants
- Lumineers or veneers not affordable

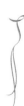
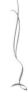

87

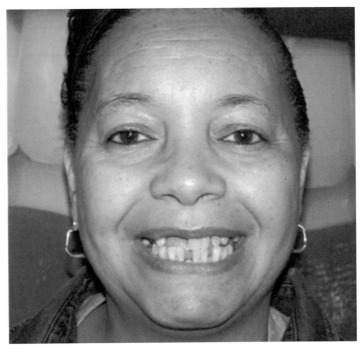

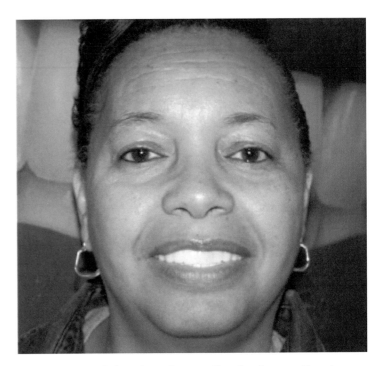

88

This patient was unhappy with her multiple missing teeth, and wanted a perfect smile for an upcoming school reunion.

After receiving her Snap-On Smile on the top and bottom, she hugged me and said, "God bless you, Dr. Z. You are a blessing." I can't tell you how great that makes me feel.

## Procedure

The process of doing a smile makeover with a Snap-On Smile is similar to applying Lumineers. In the first visit, after assessing your eligibility, you and the dentist select a style and shade. The dentist then takes an impression of your teeth. In the second visit, about three weeks later, you do a final fitting, and you can wear your Snap-On Smile home that day.

Clean your Snap-On Smile as you would your regular teeth. Your Snap-On Smile will last for three to five years and comes with a twelve month limited warranty against manufacturer's defects.

## Gum Lifts (Crown Lengthening)

In this book, I often stress the importance of good oral hygiene and regular dental vis-

its. While it is true that this is the best way to keep your gums looking pink and healthy, these practices have no effect upon the *shape* of your gums, which goes a long way to determining how good your smile looks. In this section, we will discuss the cosmetic treatments available for people who are unsatisfied with their gum lines.

Just like crooked, uneven teeth, a low, crooked gum line can mar the appearance of your smile. An even gum line is harmonious and aesthetically pleasing, and these days more people than ever are having gum lifts as part of their smile makeover. A gum lift can correct the appearance of the gums by evening the gum line and giving the appearance of longer, more symmetrical teeth (which is why the procedure is also known as crown lengthening).

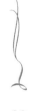

### *Reasons for a Gum Lift*

- Low gum line (which creates a "gummy" smile)
- Crooked gum line

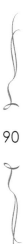

90

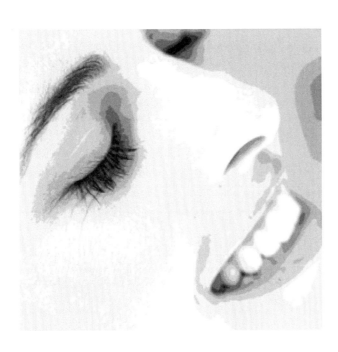

### *Procedure*

Some people cringe at the idea of cutting into their sensitive gum tissue, but in reality the procedure is quite simple, and with today's technology, healing takes place faster than ever. Traditional gum lifts are performed with a scalpel. The dentist administers a local anesthetic and cuts away at the excess gum tissue. This method of treatment is more painful and can require up to six weeks recovery. However, as with many other procedures, the painful methods of the past are no longer necessary thanks to modern technology. In our office, we use a laser to perform the treatment. In addition to being more accurate, the laser cauterizes as it lifts, resulting in much quicker healing, and excellent results, as shown on the next page.

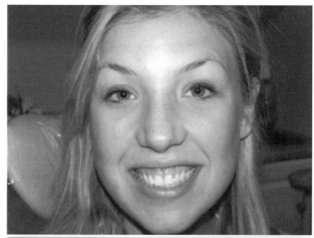

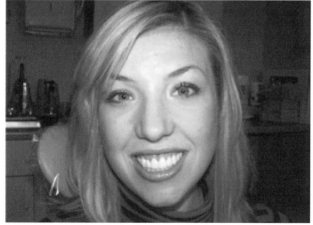

Gum contouring with a laser minimizes appearance of a gummy smile.

Following a laser gum lift, you should be back to normal in only a few days. You can speed along your recovery by observing the following practices:

- Rinse with mouthwash and/or warm saltwater twice a day.

- Avoid brushing the surgical area for twelve hours following procedure, and afterward use a soft-bristled toothbrush.

- Refrain from smoking for approximately one week following the treatment.

- If there is any bleeding or excessive swelling, contact your dentist.

## Botox and Fillers

As our lips serve to *frame* our teeth—this allows us another way to enhance one's smile.

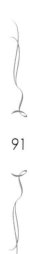

91

As you see in the pictures below, this patient had thin lips.

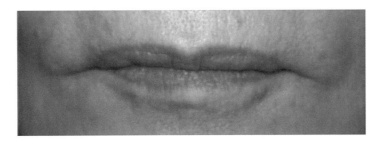

We were able to put cosmetic filler in the lips, giving them greater volume and a more youthful appearance (we tend to lose volume with age).

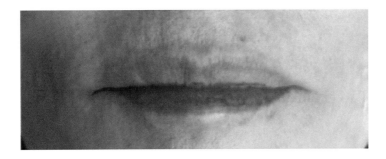

Additionally as we age, our skin loses some elasticity, creating small lines in our face. Botox can be used to relax small lines that may appear around the mouth. Not only that, we can also use Botox to decrease the downward angulation of the corners of the mouth, by relaxing the mentalis muscle that can otherwise pull down the lower lip and give a frowning appearance.

# CHAPTER 6

## THE IMPORTANCE OF DENTAL CHECKUPS

Even if you receive the best cosmetic dentistry available, your dental work has to be maintained, just like your teeth. You must practice proper hygiene regularly, both at home and at the dentist's office. This includes visiting your dentist at least once every six months. Otherwise, any work that you've had done will deteriorate, just as your normal teeth would.

If I've noticed one thing in my practice, it's that *happier people tend to take better care of themselves*. It's absolutely true. They show up for maintenance visits right on schedule. They follow up on any suggestions we make to enhance their health. They floss more. They tend to have fewer cavities.

They're more proactive in their health, and they tend to have better-looking smiles. The happier they are, the healthier they are, and the healthier they are, the happier they are. That's a good cycle to get into. Whenever they do have a problem, they treat it when it's a small problem, before it becomes difficult to manage. For example, they treat a cavity before it requires a root canal. This makes sense not only for their health but also for their pocketbook, since invasive procedures are much more costly.

There are many reasons to visit your dentist regularly:

- Brighten your smile by removing surface stains
- Prevent tooth loss from gum disease (gingivitis and the more progressive periodontitis)

93

- Prevent tooth decay by detecting cavities early
- Prevent other serious illnesses caused by gum disease
- Prevent halitosis (chronic bad breath)
- Early detection of oral pathology/oral cancer (particularly among tobacco users)
- Treat the causes of pain
- Prevent tooth loss
- Detect oral herpes/lesions of the mouth
- Prevent diabetes/heart attack (which can occur as bacteria from gum disease in the mouth makes its way into the bloodstream)

94

As you can see, these reasons extend far beyond cosmetics, yet too many people maintain the belief that a regimen of brushing alone is adequate to maintain oral health. To maintain oral health, it is necessary to go to the dentist for a checkup and cleaning *at least twice a year*. This is a bare minimum. It may even be necessary to go up to four times a year, depending on the amount of plaque on your teeth. This is affected by various factors, such as the content of your saliva and the thoroughness of your brushing/flossing. Even if you have a high-quality electric toothbrush, you won't be able to get under the gum line, as a dentist can.

We've already touched on the miracles modern cosmetic dentistry can do with your smile, and in turn your life. We've discussed how aligning your teeth can not only make them look better, but can also prevent other problems, such as TMJ dysfunction. We've also discussed the advantages of having a bright, healthy smile. However, even though people know they should be going to the dentist, they often put it off, making all kinds of excuses for why they don't go. Strangely, some are reluctant because they are afraid we'll see something wrong with their teeth. Of course, if they think about this even just a little, they'll realize that these problems aren't going away by themselves, and it would be much better to discover them early on. Other people are tentative because they believe cleanings are uncomfortable. Still others have never even *seen* a dentist. *Ever.* Why? Lifelong fear—not only of the treatment they'll receive, but of what we will find in their mouths. As you might imagine, some of it is pretty shocking. However, you'd be surprised how often all they need is a good cleaning. But they put it off, sometimes for years.

Many people still think of the dentist's office as a place that can be a bit scary and even painful. Yet advances in today's dentistry have really changed all that. Once people see what modern dentistry can do—how today's technology and methods make dentistry practically painless—that fear drops away. Some of them even laugh at themselves, literally laugh out loud, for being so scared for so long. (Often I think they're laughing out of relief.) They even start bringing in their friends, who are just as nervous as they used to be. It's like they're part of some kind of club. Admittedly, if your dentist is not up to date on the available technologies, your fears may be justified. That's why in my office, we always use the latest in technological advances. Let's look at some of these now.

## Dispelling Common Fears

In this section we will look at some common concerns about visiting the dentist and the

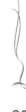

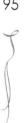

95

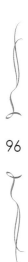

ways modern dentists address these concerns.

### *"Cleanings are uncomfortable!"*

The thought of a hygienist using a pointed metal instrument to scrape away tartar and plaque makes many patients uneasy. Trust me, dentists and hygienists know this well. There is a reason that stress levels are notoriously high among dentists. Imagine having a job where no one wants to see you because they are afraid you will hurt them, and every moment you're with them they stare at you with wide-eyed panic, expecting something to go wrong at any second.

Let's get one thing clear right away: the reason most people experience swollen and bleeding gums in the dentist's chair is that they are not coming to the dentist at least twice a year nor being thorough in their at-home brushing. Often they will come to the dentist and then never come back because of the discomfort they feel in the chair. They usually brush their teeth less as well, since they think their bleeding gums are a sign that they are brushing incorrectly. However, they should be doing the exact opposite: the more they brush their teeth, and the more they come to the dentist for regular cleanings, the more healthy and resilient their gums will become.

Dentists can do their part to make the experience as comfortable as possible for the patient. One way is to explain each step to the patient during treatment and to allow the patient to proceed at his or her own pace. This gives the patient a sense of control over the situation. The dentist may also offer medication, such as Xanax or Valium, to calm the patient's nerves. One of the best ways we've discovered to put patients at ease is to distract them with comforts, such as TVs, video games, and massage chairs. We believe that a visit to the dentist should be a pleasurable experience, which is why we refer to ourselves as a *dental spa*. Just as hotels offer more than just a bed to sleep in, dental offices today offer many amenities to make you as comfortable as possible during your visit. If yours doesn't, there should be others in your area who will.

We also do our part by using the latest in dental technology. In our office we use *ultrasonic cleaning*. Also called a sonicater, this cleaning device uses a small water-cooled tip that vibrates gently yet thoroughly across the teeth, removing tartar and plaque above and below the gum line. This creates less need for the scraping (also known as *scaling*) that many patients associate with teeth cleaning. The same process is used to clean delicate items, such as fine jewelry and watch parts, and doesn't require any special cleaning solutions—simple water is sufficient. The mechanism by which this works is somewhat complicated, but here is a short explanation: When the device is turned on, it creates vibrating waves of energy, or ultrasonic waves. These in turn create high-energy bubbles, which surround the tooth and gently but effectively remove plaque buildup from its surface. There is no scraping and no chance of injuring the gums.

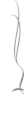

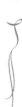

97

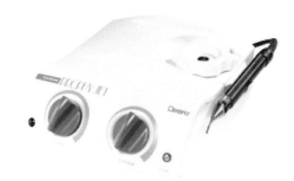

Ultrasonic Cleaner

I have used this process for years and have found it to be just as effective as traditional scaling—but a heck of a lot more comfortable for the patient.

### *"I'm afraid of needles!"*

Many patients have an exaggerated fear of needles. Even the thought of a needle in their mouth makes them cringe, as they remember the painful sting they felt during previous injections. Let's get one thing straight: that "sting" or "pinch" they felt was not even from the needle—it was from the anesthetic fluid in the needle pushing its way into the gum tissue. When anesthetic is administered properly, this pain is completely unnecessary. Previously, this was as much an art as it was a science. Fortunately, today we have tools that take the guesswork out of the process. In my office, we have a device called

"The Wand." The Wand is a machine that controls the flow and pressure of the anesthetic coming through the needle (previously Novocain, but increasingly dentists today are using Lidocaine). Rather than manipulating the pressure of the injection manually by hand, the Wand precisely controls the amount and speed of the fluid coming out through the needle. It maintains the pressure at such a low level that it's virtually painless to the patient. It also happens to have a nonthreatening appearance, shaped much like a pencil.

In addition to the Wand, there are other ways dentists can lessen the pain of injections. These include offering nitrous oxide to patients before injections and applying a topical anesthetic to the gums before the needle is inserted (however, again, it usually is not the needle itself that causes most of the discomfort).

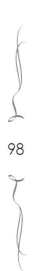

98

## *"Dental surgery is painful and scary!"*

Any surgery is a frightening proposition, yet for many patients, the thought of cutting into one's gums produces a visceral sense of horror, making their skin crawl. This is another case where patients' fears can be alleviated by state-of-the-art technology: lasers. In many cases, instead of using scalpels, I can use a laser. A laser allows the dentist to perform oral surgery using no metal cutting tool whatsoever. Not only is it less painful for the patient, but the laser even sutures (closes) veins at the same time that it cuts. It cauterizes as it cuts, stopping the bleeding immediately. What does that mean for the patient? It means less edema and swelling, and less downtime during healing.

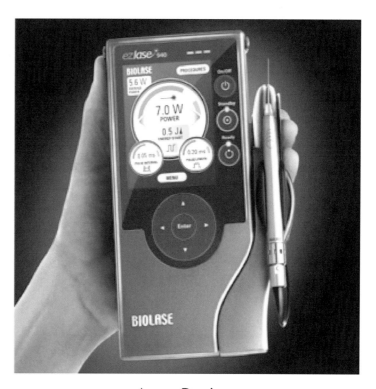

Laser Device
Biolase Technology, Inc.

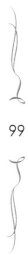

99

Interestingly, laser dentistry is not a recent development. It's actually been available since the early 1990s, but according to the Academy of Laser Dentistry, fewer than 10 percent of dentists in the United States use it. That's truly a surprisingly low amount, especially since many professionals consider this technology to be the future of dentistry. I've found my patients are eager to try it. It's less intimidating than traditional surgical approaches, and the procedure is fairly painless. Also, traditional surgical procedures using metal tools likely require a Novocain shot to numb the mouth, whereas laser dentistry usually only requires a topical cream anesthetic. Plus, as I said earlier, incisions heal faster, because the laser cauterizes as it cuts.

The treatment is also appealing for those children who need their gums reshaped around their braces, which is a fairly common problem. Since children usually aren't as diligent about performing dental hygiene, their gums can begin to grow over braces. For these children, the laser is not only the less scary option, but it is actually kind of appealing, since they associate lasers with images from science fiction movies. They're often excited that I use such a "futuristic" tool in the dentist's office.

I treated the girl mentioned earlier who had developed a form of gingivitis due to her inability to properly floss and brush while wearing metal braces. I used a laser to contour her gums and remove the excess tissue without the need for anesthetics or shots. The results of this can be seen in these before and after pictures.

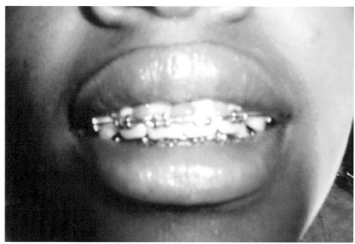

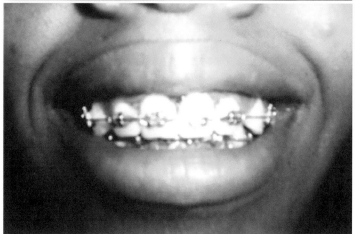

I've also used the laser to perform surgery on children born with tongue-tie (ankyloglossia), a congenital condition marked by an unusually short and thick frenulum, the membrane that connects the underside of the tongue to the floor of the mouth. This condition can decrease the mobility of the tongue and inhibit one's speech, causing a lisp. It can also affect the health of the teeth and gums, since the tongue is unable to sweep across the mouth as it should to clear excess saliva and food debris. This may lead to cavities and/or gingivitis.

Normally, a lingual frenectomy would be performed to treat this condition. This involves clamping the frenum, snipping away its leading edge, and then stitching it up. This requires a local anesthetic and can be done at your dentist's office. Afterward, it can take from a few days up to a few weeks to heal, which can be a painful process, requiring careful eating and frequent rinsing with a saline solution. With a laser, the procedure is much simpler. It takes just twenty minutes, after which the patient can move their tongue freely. Many speech therapists send their clients to us to help with this condition. Thus, a potentially long-term and upsetting problem for a child can be solved quickly. Parents are very grateful for this simple procedure.

Of course, it's not just children and their parents who appreciate this. Not long ago, I treated a woman who was so pleased by her results—as well as the ease and comfort of the procedure—that she drove an hour and a half each way to see me rather than visit a closer dentist. She claims it was worth it.

I also use the laser to perform gum lifts in cases where a patient has a gummy smile (see chapter 5 for more on gum lifts). With the laser, I can make their gums look perfect in half an hour. I've even used the laser for periodontal disease (gum disease). I can aim it in the pockets and it kills the bacteria in the pockets and cleans them. I can also use a laser for many root canals—and do a better job than I would with a traditional drill. Additionally, I've excised lesions with a laser, removing overgrowth of tissue.

### "X-rays will give me radiation poisoning!"

Unlike the others, this concern does not involve pain or discomfort. X-rays are painless. However, people are concerned with the effects they may have on their body. The good news is that there have been great advances in X-ray machine technology, reducing the amount of radiation the subject is exposed to. Lately there has been much ado about exposure to radiation, thanks to sensational stories in the news about the use of backscatter technology in airports and nuclear catastrophe in Japan. While radiation exposure is no doubt a serious issue, thankfully there is nothing to worry about when it comes to dental X-rays. These days, a typical dose of radiation received in the dentist's chair would be less than what you would get on a long-distance flight. Even the lead aprons traditionally used to protect the patient are no longer necessary with modern X-rays; today, they are provided more for the patient's peace of mind than for any sound medical reason.

The latest X-ray advancement is digital radiography. In this procedure, digital images are used in place of photographic film to produce a more detailed image of the mouth, quickly and without the use of chemical processing. The pictures come out as well as any conventional X-rays, but with *much less* radiation exposure to the patient. I can even display the pictures on a TV monitor for the patient, in addition to printing hardcopy photographs.

Speaking of displays, there's been another advancement that benefits the patient: intraoral cameras. These are tiny cameras—about the size and shape of an electric toothbrush—that the dentist inserts into the mouth. It can also display on a TV monitor in the exam room, and it prints photographs as well. So now I don't just tell a patient that they have a cavity—I show them up close. The patient can see exactly what I'm talking about, which takes away some of the mystery—and the fear.

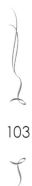

103

### *"The dentist makes me gag!"*

Of course, you don't always need technology to make the patient more comfortable. Sometimes all you need is a little knowledge. I had one patient who was hesitant to come to my office, not because she anticipated pain, but because she would gag anytime a dentist put his fingers into her mouth. It didn't matter how careful the dentist tried to be—she would gag every time. This can be a traumatic experience for anyone who suffers from this problem. There is a sense of complete loss of bodily control, similar to the sense of drowning. The gag reflex is triggered when pressure is applied to the soft palate, where the vagus nerve is located. When the nerve is triggered, there is a convulsion in the muscles of the throat, leading to a sensation of nausea (which can lead to vomiting). Sensitivity to this pressure is highly variable among patients—some are not affected at all, while others will retch if the slightest pressure is applied, making it impossible for them to brush their back teeth, swallow pills, etc.

Fortunately, all it takes is a few simple adjustments to help with this. One is salt. Simply putting normal salt in a specific area of the mouth (on the vagus nerve) "numbs" the area and diminishes the gag reflex. In tougher cases, we can swab a topical anesthetic on the roof of the mouth, which helps cut down the gag reflex. We can administer nitrous oxide (laughing gas), which is also known to relax patients and reduce the gag reflex during dental procedures. We can have the patient sit down rather than lie flat. This works due partly to the change in position and partly to psychological reasons, as the patient feels more in control and less vulnerable when sitting up. However, the best way we can alleviate the gag reflex is by getting the work done more quickly. That's why when filling cavities we use "curing lights," which greatly shorten the time tooth fillings need to harden. I use one of the latest lights, a laser that needs to be shined over the white filling material for only five seconds to cure (harden) it. It is both quicker and easier for the patient.

By detailing many of the advancements in the field of dentistry, I hope I've dispelled the myth that treatment has to be uncomfortable. Even so, there will still be those who hesitate, still holding on to old phobias. Part of this, I'm sure, is due to the environment of the dentist's office—the familiar sights, smells, and sounds that the patient has come to associate with pain and discomfort. That's one of the reasons why I designed my office like a spa—to put people at ease and encourage them to *want* to visit me. However, my encouragement doesn't stop at getting you in the door of your dentists' office. I would

also encourage you to create a relationship with your dentist—a relationship of trust. As in all relationships, trust requires communication.

### Communicating with Your Dentist

How do you develop a relationship of trust with your dentist? First, when selecting a dentist, be honest. Tell the dentist if you have any misgivings. At the same time, clarify your expectations regarding treatments. The dentist in turn needs to be honest with you, telling you if your expectations are unrealistic. This way you can see if his philosophy fits with yours.

I'd suggest going to a few consultations with different dentists. Don't just choose the first one you meet. Some people think all dentists are more or less alike, but in reality there is great variance among dentists—in skill, in

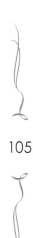

105

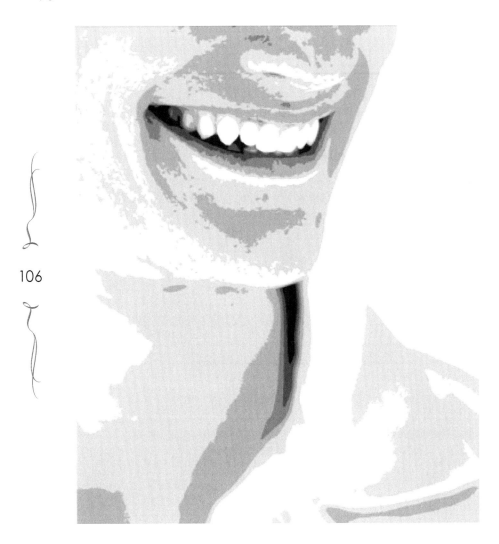

demeanor, in availability (which is important if you need emergency work done), and in knowledge. Here are a few things to look for when visiting a new dentist:

- Does he have a clean office?
- Does he have high-end technology?
- Are you comfortable with the support staff?

All this will tell you a lot about the way the doctor runs his practice. For example, if the practice is in an old building that looks slightly disheveled, then you're probably going to get that kind of dentistry.

Most importantly, once you've chosen your dentist, don't keep things to yourself. If you're not satisfied with something, tell him about it. Don't just leave unhappy. As I have said, true happiness comes from the inside. Even if you look better, if you are bottling something up inside you, it is bound to come out eventually. Your dentist won't know there's a problem—nor will he be able to change it—if you don't tell him.

As in any important relationship, communication is the key. Early on in my career, I had a patient whose teeth I restored to the ideal vision. Well, as it turns out, it was my ideal vision, but not hers. She had wanted to keep the gap between her two front teeth, although she never told me this. I had to redo the procedure to put that gap back in. That taught me the lesson that not only is communication important, but also that beauty truly is in the eye of the beholder. The patient needs to communicate and the dentist must listen. A dentist shouldn't assume a patient wants a particular type of smile, and the patient shouldn't assume the dentist knows exactly what they want.

## Tell Your Dentist Which Medications You're Taking

During any dental treatment, you must be forthcoming about any medications you are taking. Don't assume there will be no contraindications. Certain medications can affect the health and treatment of your mouth. For instance, calcium channel blockers are commonly used to treat angina. While they can help with this condition, they can also cause enlarged gums, leading to gum growth over your teeth (gingival hyperplasia). These drugs can also cause "dry mouth" (xerostomia). Both of these can be mistaken for bad hygiene if the dentist is not aware that meds are being taken. When I see this growth happening and determine it's not congenital but rather due to some medication, I will contact the patient's doctor to find if there's an alternative drug that might not produce those side effects. Likewise, if a pa-

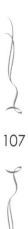

107

tient had a medical condition that required her to be on blood thinners, I would need to contact her doctor. I'd want to learn the bleeding and coagulation times for that patient, and I would want to know how much we can safely reduce her use of blood thinners before and after surgery.

Interestingly, sometime patients don't want to reveal that they're taking certain medications, such as seizure medications. I'm sure part of this is due to embarrassment, but in many cases they simply do not think it is relevant. They figure since I'm a dentist, any medication they are taking could not possibly be related to what I'm working on. But as I emphasize throughout this book, *everything is related.*

Similarly, there are patients who don't want to reveal they have hepatitis. You might think you are protecting your dignity by

withholding this information, but if you end up in the hospital because of medications I've prescribed you (e.g., Motrin), you'll feel more foolish than dignified. I had a patient for several years that I'd come to know fairly well. At a certain point, I needed to give her some painkillers. She had filled out her medical forms like everyone does. For various reasons, I suspected she wasn't being completely honest with me, and I questioned if what she had filled out was accurate. Ultimately, I asked her directly if she'd ever had hepatitis. She became uncomfortable but continued to deny it. But it was critical that I find out, so I called her MD, and sure enough she was being treated for hepatitis. Sparing her the embarrassment of telling her, I quietly changed to a different painkiller that would be safe for her to take. Clearly she was embarrassed to reveal this to me. However, if I'm your doctor, it's just not in your best interest to keep medical secrets from me. Please keep that in mind for your dentist as well.

Ultimately, you will want a dentist that you trust. This way, you'll also be receptive to any suggestions they make. For example, if a dentist that you trust suggests a night guard after putting on Lumineers, then you should get the night guard and use it. (A night guard is a mouthpiece for patients who tend to grind their teeth; they wear it while sleeping so they don't damage their Lumineers.) If you don't listen to him—if you feel you got the smile you wanted and don't want to do anything more—then you'll likely ruin your terrific smile. Similarly, with Invisalign, once you've straightened your teeth, you will need to wear the retainer that the dentist suggests. Otherwise, your teeth will shift and you'll be back to square one. The same idea applies to maintaining your teeth. If you don't come in for cleanings as often as you're encouraged to, your teeth will suffer the consequences of that as well.

Let your dentist be the expert in their field, just as you trust experts in other professions. Listen to what they have to say. That, of course, requires trust, and it requires you making your concerns known. We dentists have many highly developed skills, but they usually don't include mindreading. So help us to help you.

109

# CHAPTER 7

## CARING FOR YOUR TEETH

In the previous chapter, we talked about maintaining your smile through regular dental checkups. However, this is only the tip of the iceberg when it comes to dental care and oral hygiene. Typically, you will only see the dentist twice a year. The other 363 days, *you* are in control of your dental health. In order to maintain your fabulous new smile, you need to exercise proper oral hygiene and dental care every single day. In this chapter, we will discuss some of the fundamentals of home dental care. Following this, we will discuss some of the bad habits that people have when it comes to their teeth.

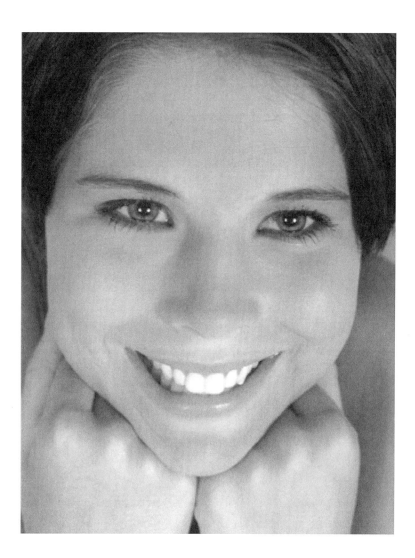

### *Oral Hygiene: Your Daily Routine*

Let's make one thing clear from the beginning. Despite all the products offered at your local pharmacy—the gels, rinses, picks, and other devices—your oral care ultimately depends upon performing two basic tasks: *brushing* and *flossing*. While these other treatments can certainly enhance your oral care, your oral health will depend on *how frequently* and *how well* you brush and floss.

### Brushing

Regular, proper brushing is the cornerstone of any oral health regimen. The goal of brushing is to remove plaque from the gum line and to sweep bacteria out of the mouth, reducing the chance of cavities and oral infections. I recommend brushing twice every day, and after every time you eat sugary foods. It doesn't matter so much which toothpaste you use. What does matter is your *frequency* and your *technique*.

**Technique:** Toothpaste manufacturers make all sorts of promises when it comes to removing plaque, tartar, and bacteria. The amount of plaque and bacteria you remove has little to do with the toothpaste you choose and everything to do with your technique. In my experience, most people could stand to improve their brushing skills. Here are some tips:

- Brush every surface of your teeth, every time you brush.

- Focus on the gum line, holding the bristles at a 45-degree angle and pushing softly toward the gums.

- Use soft, circular motions, sweeping and rolling away from the gum line.

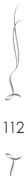

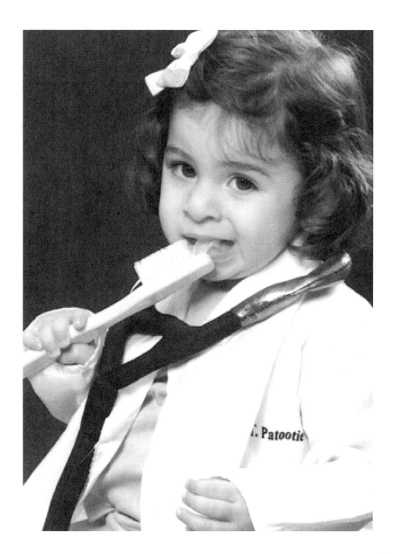

- Don't rush: spend about ten seconds in each area, for a total of about two minutes.

**Choosing a toothbrush:** There is a wide selection of brushes available at your local pharmacy. It's easy to become distracted by the variety of sizes, brands, and designs available, but really, there are only two key considerations:

- *Buy a toothbrush with the softest bristles you can find.* Toothbrushes with hard bristles can cause abrasions to the enamel and recession of the gum line over time.

- *Change your toothbrush/toothbrush head often (every three to six months).* How long your toothbrush lasts will depend on the quality of the toothbrush and how aggressively you brush your teeth. Once the bristles show any signs of flaring, it is

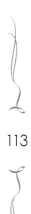

113

time to change your brush. Toothbrushes with frayed bristles are not as effective, and they are more prone to picking up bacteria, which can cause infections.

### Electric or Manual?

Whether you use an electric or manual toothbrush is mainly a matter of personal preference. While an electric toothbrush rotates and oscillates for you, effectively removing plaque, you are perfectly capable of replicating this motion with a manual toothbrush. In addition, because of their wider surface area, manual toothbrushes do a better job of brushing the tongue. Brushing the tongue is important, both for fresh breath and for removing bacteria in general. Unfortunately, electric toothbrushes do a poor job of cleaning the tongue. A good practice is to keep both types of toothbrush in your house, using each one according to how you feel at the

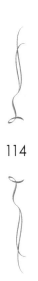

114

time. If you feel your teeth need a vigorous cleaning, use the electric toothbrush. If you want to clean your entire mouth, reach for the manual toothbrush. With both types of brush, the most important consideration is the condition of the brush head. Again, be sure to replace the brush head every three to six months.

### Flossing

Flossing is extremely important. Dental floss gets into the spaces between your teeth where a toothbrush cannot reach, removing food particles that would turn into sugar and erode the enamel and cause cavities. In my own practice, most of the cavities I see are between the teeth, which means that *most patients coming in to the dentist to treat cavities are coming in because they are not flossing*. In fact, flossing may even be more important than brushing.

I advise patients to floss twice a day, immediately after brushing. Make it part of your normal routine. If you are prone to bleeding gums, this is most likely happening because you have some sort of gingivitis, which is happening because you are not flossing on a regular basis. If you do experience bleeding gums, do not let that deter you from flossing; this will stop once your gums become more healthy and resilient.

## Respecting Your Teeth

Just about all the cosmetic procedures we've discussed in this book are designed to be permanent, but just like your teeth, they are only permanent for as long as you take care of them. If you mistreat your teeth,

through either *neglect* or *abuse*, then all your good dental work could be undone.

As with all life experiences, what we're exposed to can change who we are. Some exposures can do great harm over a lifetime. In our lives, we are continually exposed to harmful substances in our environment, what some call "environmental exposures." Pollution and chemicals are part of our world, and that is unlikely to change in the foreseeable future. Certainly we can make choices to limit some of our exposures, like choosing healthier cleaning products in our homes. But we also should focus on making our bodies as strong and healthy as possible, with robust immune systems capable of fending off damaging exposures and illnesses. That will lead us to happier lives.

But some people make choices that unnecessarily expose their teeth and gums to stress,

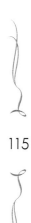

115

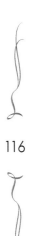

sometimes dramatically shortening the lives of their teeth—and their lives in general.

## Tobacco

Even though its widespread use has diminished greatly, some people still smoke. It's well known by now that smoking can negatively affect us in numerous ways. What may not be so well known are the consequences it can have in our mouths—particularly our gums.

Smoking can negatively affect the teeth, but the effects are mainly cosmetic. It darkens teeth as the smoke stains the enamel, and it can also stain dental prosthesis, including Lumineers (although it is somewhat easier to remove tobacco stains from porcelain, since porcelain is less porous than dental enamel). The effect on the gums, however, is more significant. Most people don't realize that smoking interferes with our blood's cir-

culation. Blood vessels actually spasm in response to cigarette smoke, which in turn can hinder blood flow. The result: the gums end up getting an insufficient supply of blood.

Making matters worse, smokers generally don't know their actions are causing a problem with their gums, since their gums don't display the "symptom" most commonly associated with gum disease: bleeding. In fact, smokers' gums tend to bleed less than those of some nonsmokers. Why? For the same reason just described—there's insufficient blood supply traveling to the gums. By the time the problem eventually becomes known, serious damage has often resulted to the gums, because it's gone unnoticed for so long.

Oddly, some people continue to use another form of tobacco even though it is well known to cause gum problems: chewing tobacco. People who chew keep tobacco in one area of their mouth for extended periods of time. This is well documented as a potential cause of oral cancer. Even before that happens, the tissue in that area may begin to whiten, which is often an early sign of cancer. Chewing tobacco can also cause a recession of the gums in that area.

Unfortunately, tobacco is addictive. So, even armed with irrefutable knowledge, it's still hard for some people to change their habits. The best bet: don't start using it in the first place.

## Hard Objects

I encounter people taking their teeth for granted every day—not only through improper care or lack of regular dental visits, but also in the way they use them. Teeth are meant for eating. Yes, they look nice. Yes,

they affect how our words sound. But their primary purpose is for eating. Yet some people use them as tools. They use them to open food packages, bite off clothing tags, even open beer bottles (yes, really!). Then they are surprised when they break their teeth. While teeth are strong, they have limitations. Our bones are strong too, but we know that they can break. At a certain angle and a certain stress point, you can break anything. People need to recognize front teeth may only be an eighth of an inch thick. They are supposed to be used for one reason only—cutting and chewing food.

Once someone breaks a tooth, they'll likely need a crown. After this, they usually don't take them for granted again. It's a lesson learned the hard way. Here are some general guidelines for what not to put in your mouth. The same advice applies to every-

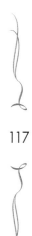

117

118

one, whether you have had cosmetic dentistry or not.

- Don't use your teeth as a tool.

- Don't bite your nails.

- Don't open packages—even ripping a bag of chips can apply shearing forces that can crack teeth.

- Don't use your teeth to open cans of soda.

- Don't chew ice.

- Don't crack seeds or nuts with your front teeth. Even cracking sunflower seeds can cause small chips in the front teeth; also, the salt can erode the enamel.

## *Vomiting/Bulimia*

While maintaining a healthy body weight is critical to our good health, our media has helped turn our desire to be thin into a dangerous obsession. I've come across some people who try to keep their weight down by throwing up. *On purpose.* That is not a healthy way to lose weight overall, and it is particularly harmful to our teeth. Essentially, they're causing chemical erosion on their teeth. This harms the enamel and may result in teeth that need root canals.

I've seen this mostly with teenage girls and young women in their early to mid-twenties who are obsessed with their weight. For me, things get more complicated when I see someone underage doing this. They may not want me to tell their mother or father, but I'm obligated by law to inform the parents because they're underage. I'm sure the parents appreciate that I inform them, but it can become awkward for the patient and me. However, by alerting their family, hopefully I'm not only helping them save their teeth, but I'm also intervening in a hidden activity that might otherwise progress into other serious health issues.

## Sugar

From the time we were very young, we've ignored the adult voices warning, "Don't eat too much sugar—it's bad for your teeth." As adults, our inner voices are more likely concerned with the calories we are consuming. Unfortunately, the temptation is strong, especially as sugar appears in more food products today than ever. It's a legitimate health hazard, but unlike cigarettes or alcohol, you don't need to be above a certain age to buy it, and there are no warning labels on it.

Perhaps there should be.

I'm not going to say never eat sugar. What would be the point? But you should recog-

nize that it really must be consumed in moderation. What makes this more challenging today is that sugar is often "hidden" in processed foods. Hidden, that is, until you read the label, which I recommend. You might be surprised—even shocked—to see how much sugar is contained in many everyday food products.

There is no doubt that sugar contributes to the creation of cavities. When sugars and other carbohydrates are eaten, bacteria in the mouth feed off them, producing acid as a waste product. This lowers the mouth's pH to below 5.7, which contributes to demineralization of tooth enamel and in turn creates potential for cavities.

But it's important to recognize that sugar has effects on other parts of the body as well— none of them good. It contributes to obesity, hyperactivity, and difficulty concentrating; it

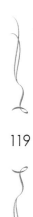

119

suppresses our immune system; it disturbs our mineral balances; and it hinders our absorption of calcium and magnesium, creating a more acidic environment in the body. It also increases cholesterol, contributes to osteoporosis and diabetes, feeds cancer cells in cancer patients, causes toxemia during pregnancy, contributes to cardiovascular disease, and even causes premature aging—especially to our skin, by altering the structure of collagen (you'd think that would be enough to deter people in our youth-obsessed society). And the list really does go on.

Will you stop eating sugar entirely? Likely not. But certainly you want to limit your intake. And if you are a parent, you should limit your children's intake so they don't get lifelong habits of seeking out sugar when they're hungry or tired or just looking for some emo-

120

tionally satisfying "comfort food." You'll be doing them a great service.

## Pass the Sugar (Substitute), Please

I give away candy. Bowls of the stuff. Mostly to children.

Am I trying to drum up repeat business? Actually, I'm doing the opposite. In fact, I was recently featured in the *Chicago Tribune* and the *Southtown Star* publications about this activity and my reasons behind doing it.

I'm serious about handing out candy to children. I do it once a year, at Halloween. Now, this is a far cry from what I used to do, which was to pay children *not* to eat their Halloween candy. I would give them five dollars for every pound they would turn in to me. I did this to prevent them from eating these holiday treats, which are often the worst kind of candy—the sticky caramel stuff that adheres to your teeth—and risk developing cavities. But I came to realize they'd still eat candy. That's what I did when I was a child—and while many things have changed since I was young, eating candy isn't one of them.

Fortunately, candy has changed.

Or at least one type of candy has, and that's what lies behind my unusual action. As a result, today dental disease can actually be *treated* with candy and chewing gum.

Sound bizarre?

It might. After all, for decades, dentists have advised us to avoid sugar. But I'm not talking about gum and candy sweetened with sugar, but with xylitol.

There are many sugar substitutes and alternatives available today, but xylitol stands out when it comes to dentistry. Xylitol is a naturally occurring sweetener found in the fibers of many vegetables, grains, and fruits, including corn husks, mushrooms, oats, and a variety of berries. Studies have shown that using xylitol (e.g., chewing xylitol gum) actually benefits teeth by decreasing the accumulation of plaque.

How?

As we discussed, when we eat sugars and other carbohydrates, the bacteria in our mouth produces acid as a by-product. This demineralizes tooth enamel and creates the potential for cavities. Xylitol is what's called a five-carbon polyol, which means that no acid is produced as a by-product of its consumption. When xylitol products are used, the pH balance in the mouth goes back above pH 5.7, reducing erosion of enamel and improving the remineralization of the teeth.

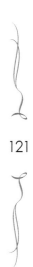

121

122

Xylitol also holds back growth of the main bacteria linked to tooth decay, *Streptococcus mutans*. These bacteria cannot utilize xylitol as an energy source. If used regularly, three to five times daily, xylitol will prevent the bacteria from multiplying, causing this bacteria to move off the plaque and into the saliva. This makes it harder for plaque to adhere to the tooth surface. Additionally, xylitol-sweetened products create an increase in the flow of saliva, which further helps prevent cavities by rinsing away excess sugar residues and neutralizing any acids that have formed.

Research now shows that chewing xylitol gum regularly after meals and snacks reduces accumulation of plaque biofilm. In fact, eating xylitol-sweetened candies over a four-day period, with no other oral hygiene, leads to a 50 percent reduction in plaque.

Today, xylitol is not used just as a sugar substitute in a variety of gums and candies. Its benefits to teeth have found their way into a variety of dental products, including dental floss, dental gels, and toothpastes, which often contain 25–36 percent xylitol in their ingredients.

## Tips for Parents of Young Children

Parents often ask me the best way to instill good dental habits in their children. I always tell them: the best way to ensure a lifetime of good oral hygiene is to start early.

The American Academy of Pediatrics recommends taking your child to see the dentist for the first time when he or she is around twelve months old. This is to get them comfortable with visiting a dentist. I will make their visit fun by giving them a gentle "ride" as they sit in the exam chair by moving it up and down, letting them look in a mirror while I count their teeth with them (as I also look for cavities), and even let them put on a little mask like mine or try on a pair of our plastic gloves if they like.

As they get older and come in for regular appointments, we will educate them more about their teeth and how they can help care for them at home. There are still things that parents can do to help make this experience even easier for the child. You can encourage children by telling them how big they are now and how they can now go to the dentist like Mom and Dad. You can make it seem like a visit to a friend rather than a scary medical treatment. You can also get them excited by telling them about all the cool things at the dentist's office—like the lasers! This usually gets my young patients interested. However, the best way to get them into a good oral care routine is to

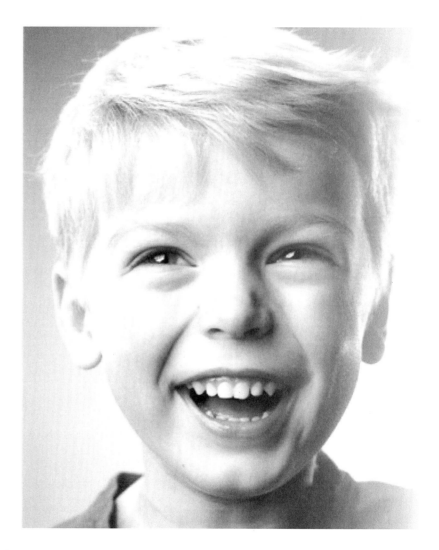

123

124

practice it from an early age *at home*. Start by teaching them good brushing, flossing, and dietary habits when they are small—beginning around two years old. Get them excited about brushing by making a game out of it, seeing who can brush fastest or longest. You can also buy them a toothbrush featuring a favorite cartoon character. The point is to make it fun and not like an arduous task. Then as they mature, you can modify your approach to encourage their using the proper brushing technique (which we also will show them in our office).  And of course, never make a punishment out of brushing their teeth or going to the dentist (e.g., "If you don't stay quiet, I'll take you to the dentist"). I know I shouldn't have to tell people that, but you'd be surprised.

## Other tips:

- Don't use candy as a reward for good behavior. This can lead to bad habits later.

- Starting at birth, clean your child's gums using a wet cloth. Progress to a soft bristled pediatric toothbrush when the first tooth erupts.

- Begin flossing your child's teeth at about four years of age. (They likely won't develop the muscular coordination to floss by themselves until they are eight to ten years old.)

- Before the child is seven years old, you should put only a pea-sized amount of toothpaste on their brush. Toothpaste may seem "hot" or "spicy" to a toddler, so you don't want to overdo it.

## Baby Bottles

On the other hand, sometimes it's the *parents* that are the source of a problem for their children's teeth. For instance, some parents let their babies go to sleep while sucking on a baby bottle. They do this to comfort the sleeping baby, and in turn to make it easier on the parent. But this may end up causing "baby bottle tooth decay" (as milk and juice, the most common drinks given to toddlers, are naturally full of carbohydrates). In their efforts to ensure their child is rested (and let's be honest, to get a little more sleep themselves), these parents may be harming their children's teeth.

## Baby Teeth Are Important

I know some parents give children candy to calm them down. But the reality is they aren't calming them. They're putting more sugar in their bodies and the children are becoming more hyperactive. At the same time, they're putting sugar on their teeth, which can be a big contributor to cavities.

Part of the problem is the belief among many parents that "It's just a baby tooth. They're going to fall out anyway and be replaced. We don't have to worry about them."

But that isn't true. *It's very important that the baby teeth remain healthy and intact.* They create pathways for adult teeth. If you have a missing baby tooth, or a tooth that must be extracted because of severe decay, then the pathway for the adult tooth to come out will be disrupted. The adult tooth won't have the *resistance* it would have had trying to pushing out the baby tooth. So the adult tooth comes through much earlier than it's supposed to. Now the growth pattern is changed, and this may cause your child to

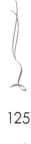

125

need braces in the future when otherwise they may not have.

But leaving a bad baby tooth in the mouth isn't a solution either. The cavity in the baby tooth can actually get to the adult tooth underneath and develop there. So by the time the new adult tooth comes out, it already has a cavity—and potentially a large one, as it's had all that time to grow unobserved.

Baby teeth need to be taken care of—just like the baby.

# CHAPTER 8

## PREVENTING GUM DISEASE

Our bodies are astonishing biological creations, with astonishingly interconnected systems. That is how we can run, create, build, speak, and even repair ourselves.

Yet it is equally amazing how many of us still view different medical conditions in various parts of our body as independent from each other—as if they were separate from the rest of our body.

In regards to my own field of dentistry, many people still believe that a cavity or gum problem is a local problem. They focus simply on the condition as it affects that tooth or the gum. But these conditions can not only negatively affect other teeth and the rest of the mouth, they can affect the rest of the body as well.

There seems to be a belief that our mouth is somehow "separate" from the rest of our body, which is further fueled by the fact that we have a specialist doctor who deals primarily with the mouth—the dentist. This leads to a dangerous disconnect in the way people think about their oral health. For example, most people are aware that a blood clot in the leg could travel to the heart or lungs and lead to a serious condition. It's unlikely anyone would say, "I'm not worried about that clot. It's only in my foot." However, people lack the same awareness when it comes to their teeth and gums.

A strong correlation has been recognized between gum disease and heart disease. It has also been shown that pregnant women can experience premature births due to peri-

odontal disease. Studies have even found that more serious periodontal problems can exacerbate conditions like diabetes.

Of course, most people think that they're taking care of their gums only to preserve their teeth. Certainly having to replace a tooth due to gum disease isn't on anyone's wish list. Still, implants, although expensive, will get you your tooth back. But gum disease can have much deeper, more insidious effects, draining our overall physical health and available energy.

Let me explain how all this works.

We all know that when we get a cut on our finger or leg, we want to clean out the wound as best we can so germs don't enter the bloodstream and travel throughout the body. The same principle applies to chronically bleeding gums—even if that bleeding is minor.

128

Now, you might say, "I'm not putting dirt or germs into my mouth, so what's the problem?"

The problem is that you *are* frequently putting foreign substances in your mouth—usually three times a day at least. Food. Even if it is all healthy food, what do you think happens if food particles touch this "open wound" or possibly even get trapped in it? Over a relatively short period, that food commences to decay. In a little while, those minor bleeding gums can turn into a much larger infection.

Now you still might be saying to yourself, "Sure, that's a problem. But isn't that just a problem in the mouth?"

True, that's where it starts. But that blood in the mouth's blood vessels then travels all over the body. In fact, the vessels in the mouth are so connected to the rest of the body that some medicines and vitamin supplements (a common one is B-12) are administered by putting them under your tongue (or "sublingually"). They are efficiently absorbed into the bloodstream from there, even though there are no cuts or wounds, and transported through the body. If you have an *actual* wound, such as bleeding gum tissues from periodontal disease, that "local infection" will travel along as well as your blood passes throughout your body. Now your body's veins and organs are suddenly subject to infection as well.

One of our main concerns is how this "roaming" infection can affect the heart and circulatory system. It certainly can infect the heart, but it can also affect the arteries. How?

Here's something you may not have known: just about every illness involves inflammation. This inflammation is often a response to an infection, such as the one I'm describing now. You've undoubtedly seen inflammation result from an infected cut to your skin. An infection in the heart can cause a swelling in its tissue as well. This infection can also inflame the veins and arteries. The heart has to work harder to pump blood if the veins and arteries are obstructed due to inflammation or if the heart itself is compromised. If these conditions persist (as they can with heart disease), then the heart begins to have to work too hard to do its job. Eventually, serious problems can arise.

This is merely one condition that can arise from inflammation. But it doesn't need to be an example as dramatic as heart disease to demonstrate how a periodontal infection can affect your health. It could be something as simple as having colds more frequently or for longer periods. Or it may seem as if something is always wrong with you. You solve one

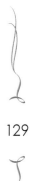

129

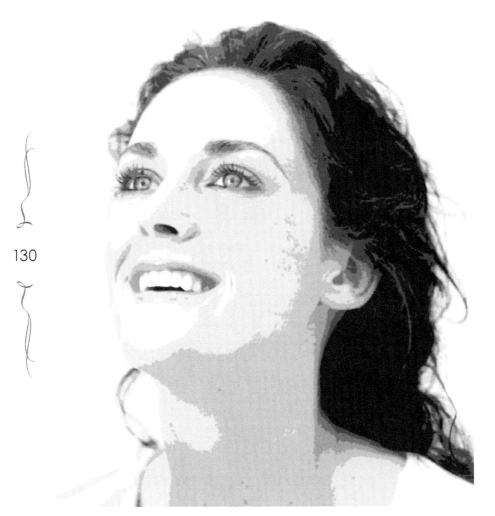

130

problem and another one surfaces. Why? Because your immune system is compromised. Any time you get an infection, your immune system tries to counter it. Each infection puts a little more strain on your immune system. Too many infections—or infections that arise chronically (like those caused continually by gum disease)—will eventually compromise the immune system to some degree. Over time, your immune system may not be able to perform its primary task adequately, leading to a life-threatening illness.

Another problem with gum disease is that it usually isn't painful. Unless you know what to look for, or a dentist catches it, you may not know you have it. But as the immune system is busy fighting off unnecessary infections, your health may be compromised in small ways. You might feel more tired in general. You might have less stamina playing sports and get winded faster. You might sleep poorly. Your digestion may seem off. You may not be able to focus at work like you used to. You just don't feel as great, and as a result, you won't feel as happy. Eventually, even your smile might suffer. (Were you wondering when I'd get back to that?) Reducing infections not only improves your health, it increases your vitality—your zest for life! It can improve your outlook—and your smile.

The good news? It doesn't take a lot of effort to correct gum disease. When I see patients, my first objective is to remove this source of infection in their bodies. Then I can work at improving the appearance of their teeth.

Despite our knowledge, many dentists still don't place enough emphasis on this issue. They may even still look at gum disease as a local problem. But don't let that stop you. Be your own best advocate. Find out from your dentist (or another one if yours remains unresponsive) what you can do to fix and prevent gum disease. Once you do, you may find your other health problems diminish. You may even discover you have more energy and a more positive outlook on life.

And then we all benefit as well—as you begin sharing your beautiful smile with us more than even before. Hopefully you're seeing why it's so important to get your teeth and gums professionally cleaned regularly, at least every six months.

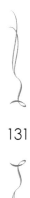

## Gum Diseases and Treatments

Periodontal disease is diagnosed by your dentist or dental hygienist during a periodontal examination. This type of exam should always be part of your regular dental checkup.

131

A periodontal probe (small dental instrument) is gently used to measure the sulcus (pocket or space) between the tooth and the gums. The depth of a healthy sulcus measures three millimeters or less and does not bleed. The periodontal probe helps indicate if pockets are deeper than three millimeters. As periodontal disease progresses, the pockets usually get deeper. If periodontal disease is found, your dentist or hygienist will use pocket depths, amount of bleeding, inflammation, tooth mobility, etc., to categorize the severity.

### Gingivitis

Gingivitis is the first stage of periodontal disease. Plaque and its toxic by-products irritate the gums, making them tender, inflamed, and likely to bleed.

### Periodontitis

Plaque hardens into calculus (tartar). As calculus and plaque continue to build up, the gums begin to recede from the teeth. Deeper pockets form between the gums and teeth and become filled with bacteria and pus. The gums become very irritated and inflamed, and they bleed easily. Slight to moderate bone loss may be present.

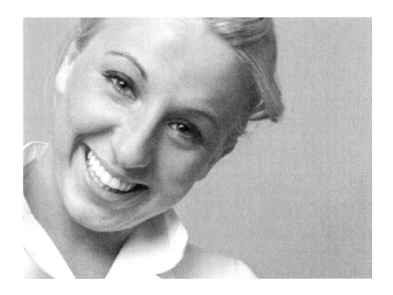

### Advanced Periodontitis

The teeth lose more support as the gums, bone, and periodontal ligaments continue to be destroyed. Unless treated, the affected teeth will become very loose and may be lost. Generalized moderate to severe bone loss may be present.

### Treatment

Periodontal treatment methods depend upon the type and severity of the disease. Your dentist and dental hygienist will evaluate you for periodontal disease and recommend appropriate treatment if needed.

Periodontal disease progresses as the sulcus (pocket or space) between the tooth and gums gets filled with bacteria, plaque, and tartar, causing irritation to the surrounding tissues. When these irritants remain in the pocket space, they can cause damage to the gums and, eventually, the bone that supports the teeth!

If the disease is caught in the early stages of gingivitis, and no damage has been done, one to two regular cleanings will be recommended. You will also be given instructions on improving your daily oral hygiene habits and having regular dental cleanings.

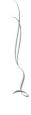

133

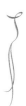

If the disease has progressed to more advanced stages, a special periodontal cleaning, called *scaling and root planing* (deep cleaning), will be recommended. It is usually done one quadrant of the mouth at a time while the area is numb. In this procedure, tartar, plaque, and toxins are removed from above and below the gum line (*scaling*) and rough spots on root surfaces are made smooth (*planing*). This procedure helps gum tissue to heal and pockets to shrink. Medications, special medicated mouth rinses, and an electric toothbrush may be recommended to help control infection and promote healing.

If the pockets do not heal after scaling and root planning, periodontal surgery may be needed to reduce pocket depths, making teeth easier to clean. Your dentist may also recommend that you see a periodontist (specialist of the gums and supporting bone).

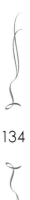

134

## *Maintenance*

It only takes twenty-four hours for plaque that is not removed from your teeth to turn into calculus (tartar)! Daily home cleaning helps control plaque and tartar formation, but those hard-to-reach areas will always need special attention.

Once your periodontal treatment has been completed, your dentist and dental hygienist will recommend that you have regular maintenance cleanings (*periodontal cleanings*), usually four times a year. At these cleaning appointments, the pocket depths will be carefully checked to ensure that they are in a healthy range. Plaque and calculus that is difficult for you to remove on a daily basis will be removed from above and below the gum line.

In addition to your periodontal cleaning and evaluation, your appointment will usually include the following:

- **Examination of diagnostic X-rays (radiographs):** Review X-rays for signs of decay, tumors, cysts, and bone loss. X-rays also help determine tooth and root positions.

- **Examination of existing restorations:** Check current fillings, crowns, etc.

- **Examination of tooth decay:** Check all tooth surfaces for decay.

- **Oral cancer screening:** Check the face, neck, lips, tongue, throat, cheek tissues, and gums for any signs of oral cancer.

- **Oral hygiene recommendations:** Review and recommend oral hygiene aids as needed (electric toothbrushes, special periodontal brushes, fluorides, rinses, etc.).

- **Teeth polishing:** Remove stain and plaque that is not otherwise removed during tooth brushing and scaling.

Good oral hygiene practices and periodontal cleanings are essential to maintaining dental health and keeping periodontal disease under control!

135

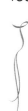

# CHAPTER 9

## SMILE FROM THE INSIDE OUT—
## WHOLE-BODY CARE

One of the "side benefits" of great health is that it makes people look even better. Certainly if you're not feeling well, your appearance suffers, even if you have the best looking teeth, makeup, hair, and clothes money can buy. We may have all of that, but if we're not feeling up to par or are sluggish, it shows.

As I proposed earlier, the real goal—in pretty much everything we do—is to increase the happiness in our lives. I know from my practice that better-looking teeth have helped many patients lead happier lives. To realize this goal, I encourage my patients to lead *healthier* lives. The human body is a fantas-

tic, complex system. It's remarkable, really. Yet we rarely think about it. When was the last time you thought about breathing? Or pumping blood through your heart? Or contracting this or that muscle to move an arm or leg?

Our body performs all kinds of functions with barely a thought from us. It can even repair itself if sick or injured. That's truly extraordinary. Sure, sometimes it needs help, but it's always making little fixes, recovering from small cuts, colds, and "misguided" meals containing too much fat, salt, and sugar. It even constantly replaces old *cells* in our body with new ones.

Most of us take all this for granted. Yet for our body to serve us, we really need to serve it as well. We can get away with a lot when we're young, but as we get older, we need to take better care of ourselves physically. It's

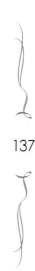

137

something we must do not just when something is wrong, but when we're feeling good also. Just like cars, our bodies need proper "maintenance." If they don't get it, something will eventually break down, requiring much more effort—and money—to fix.

I expect most of you have heard this before. After all, we live in a very health-conscious society. Health is a huge industry, with many facets. You certainly know you should eat well, exercise, and get enough sleep. But as you begin to deepen your understanding and appreciation of the amazing wonder that is your physical body, you learn that there are other things you can do to help it, some of which may not be so familiar to you.

This whole-body understanding and approach is part of what I wish to bring to you in this book. As I've said, an attractive smile

is that much more irresistible if we're feeling terrific, with plenty of energy.

## Exercise

We've all heard it: we need more exercise. As a nation, we're experiencing an epidemic of obesity, starting with our children. While this may seem to be just an attention-getting headline, the fact is that most of us are overweight and get too little exercise.

Why? For one, our diets tend to include too much fat and sugar. In addition, our lives have become busier, and we can't find time to exercise. Then "the cycle" begins: we're tired because we're not exercising enough, and we're too tired to exercise.

But your body needs to be exercised, or it will decline. Fortunately, exercise doesn't have to be incredibly strenuous or lengthy.

Even a few times a week, for twenty minutes, will do wonders. The benefits? You'll have more energy. You'll sleep better. You'll think more clearly. You'll be stronger. You'll even be thirstier (for those of you thinking the recommended amounts of water seem like a lot). You'll feel better and be happier. And it will show in your dynamic smile.

## Acupuncture

Acupuncture originated in China and can be traced back at least 2,500 years. Some even believe the earliest records of acupuncture are found in a 4,700-year-old book called *Huang Di Nei Jing* (which translates as "*Yellow Emperor's Classic of Internal Medicine*"). Believed to be the oldest medical textbook in the world, it presented theories about the heart and circulatory system

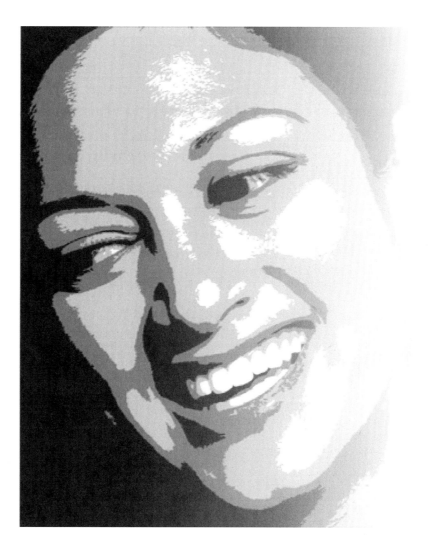

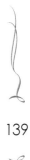

139

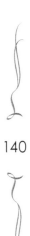

140

over 4,000 years before European medicine had any notion about them. Yet, as old as acupuncture is, most Americans had never heard of it until the early 1970s.

The basic idea of acupuncture is that there is an internal energy force called chi (pronounced *chee*). This chi is comprised of all physical, mental, emotional, and spiritual aspects of life. If the flow of this chi is insufficient, excessive, interrupted, or simply out of balance, illness can result.

The chi travels along electrical pathways in the body, called meridians. While meridians aren't visible in the same manner as blood vessels, they can become blocked.

Acupuncture is the technique of inserting very thin needles into specific points on the body and manipulating them to open up blocked energy pathways and rebalance the system. These acupuncture points are on the meridians near the skin's surface and can be accessed through needling. Some people are hesitant to try acupuncture because they are afraid the needles will hurt. But the needles are amazingly small, and, in fact, you often don't feel them at all. When you do, generally it is not because they are penetrating the skin but because they are making contact with acupuncture points and releasing blocked energy.

Interestingly, the body's response can occur near the site of the needle or in an entirely different area—just another dramatic example of how the body's areas are interconnected.

The World Health Organization and the National Institutes of Health have documented that acupuncture can help with pain relief, headaches, asthma, bronchitis, sinusitis, low back pain, osteoarthritis, carpal tunnel syndrome, tendonitis, fibromyalgia, constipation, diarrhea, spastic colon (often called irritable bowel syndrome), irregular periods, menopausal symptoms, menstrual cramps, stroke rehabilitation, urinary problems like incontinence, addictions like smoking and alcoholism, as well as post-surgery and chemotherapy-associated nausea and vomiting.

The American Academy of Medical Acupuncture adds the following to this list: sports injuries, whiplash, neck pain, sprains, sciatica, nerve pain due to compression and spinal cord injuries, allergies, tinnitus (ringing in the ears), high blood pressure, gastroesophageal or "acid" reflux (felt as heartburn or indigestion), ulcers, recurring kidney and bladder infections, premenstrual syndrome (PMS), infertility, memory problems, insomnia, multiple sclerosis, sensory disturbances, anxiety, depression, and other psychological disorders.

These long lists reflect how acupuncture meridians can affect so many areas of the body. As proof of the growing acceptance of acupuncture, an increasing number of insurance providers and HMOs cover all or part of the cost of acupuncture treatments.

As a result of its widespread effects on the body, many patients seek out acupuncture not only for specific problems they might be experiencing, but also to improve their overall energy and reduce stress. You may want to give it a try. After all, it has a history of satisfied customers going back more than 2,000 years. Maybe it can help put a cheerful smile on your face too.

## Therapeutic Massage

When we think of massage, most likely we think of soft music, scented candles, and gentle hands relaxing away our stresses of

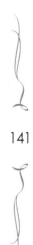

141

the day. The problem is that some of those stresses have been there a lot longer than a day.

Effective therapeutic massage not only helps you feel relaxed and rested, but also releases stored tension that may be interfering with your health and your energy flow. Yet therapeutic massage is not always comfortable. In fact, it's often not really working until it hurts.

Interestingly, therapeutic massage doesn't hurt everywhere you're touched, just in the places where you need it most. Now, most people don't usually seek out a treatment that hurts, not unless they know the benefits involved. So it helps to know that the painful locations are likely where there are stored tensions or waste products from the body.

By "waste products," I mean by-products in our bodies that have been created by living

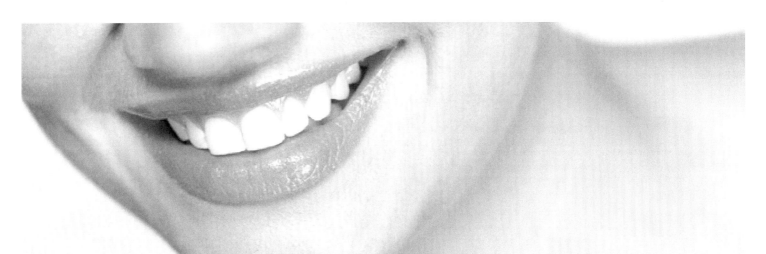

in today's contaminated world. They may be the result of what we take in—in our air, water, and food. They may have built up for a short time, like a few weeks, or may have been accumulating for years. Or they may be from stored tensions due to different kinds of stress or even from exercise.

The problem arises when they impede circulation through the body. Similar to a misaligned spine, they can inhibit blood circulation, as well as communications to various parts of the body through the nervous system. Continued unchecked, the situation can worsen, causing all sorts of problems. These problems can occur in distant areas of your body, which at first may not seem to have any connection with the areas where you might feel pain during your massage. But, as I have emphasized several times in this book, the body's various parts are interconnected.

If the therapist uses the right technique, with enough pressure, over time the treatments should help release the stored waste. The area that was hurting will no longer be so sensitive to the therapist's touch, and you should see improved energy and health in other areas too.

You may need to drink more water to help flush away the toxins as they are released. You might even feel a little worse right after treatment, as the toxins are being expelled. But that should quickly subside, and you should soon feel much better overall. Just be cautious about stopping massage therapy if you don't feel so great for those first few days following a treatment. Some people think they should instantly feel better without any additional discomfort. You might recall the oft-used phrase, "No pain, no gain." Not that I'm a believer in everything needing to hurt to be beneficial. As I've said, I make great

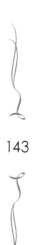

143

efforts to keep my dentistry as pain-free as possible. But in this case, the long-term improvement should outweigh the short-term discomfort.

You should end up feeling better and have significantly more energy available to you. Without enough energy, we are at a disadvantage in whatever we try to accomplish. It's harder for us to be at ease and cheerful. It's harder for us to enjoy ourselves.

144

One of the ways we keep our energy flowing is to keep our circulation flowing. In this respect, therapeutic massage can help tremendously.

## Chiropractic

In our language, we have a colorful expression used to describe a person afraid of facing challenges: "He has a weak spine." No one wants to hear that about themselves. No one wants to believe they're not up to the task of living life to the fullest.

Yet it may be a more accurate description than you thought.

When we think of spinal "injuries," we tend to think in extreme terms. We know a serious injury to the spine can result in paralysis or even death. Even a less dramatic injury—such as "throwing out one's back" by lifting or bending over in the wrong way—can debilitate us for days or weeks.

The importance of our spine is clear. It is the core that supports our body, and it also houses and shields vital nerves that connect to all of our body parts. That's why spinal injuries can be so deleterious. Since the spine plays such an integral role in our health, it doesn't take much imagination to realize that even minor injuries can have negative effects. In fact, it need not even be an "injury." Our day-to-day activities can often throw off our spine in small, unnoticed ways, causing minor dislocations to our vertebrae and disks that we may not even feel. But those dislocations can interfere with our energy flow, and in turn with our well-being and, ultimately, our happiness.

This is in addition to the overall fatigue that we may experience when our various body parts are not working optimally. Chiropractic can help open up the "nerve flow," realigning the small bones and disks of the spine and allowing the nerves to convey those essential signals. As a result, the problems that occur because of the inhibition of blood circulation and oxygen flow are diminished.

Yes, oxygen flow is also affected when our body is misaligned. Our blood transports oxygen, minerals, and other nutrients to our various body parts. If those areas are not properly supplied, they can become weakened. They then become less able to deal with viruses or stress (a huge problem in our busy, overbooked lives).

The fact is that any body parts that don't get sufficient fuel will suffer. Consider what might happen if our vital organs—such as our brain, heart, lungs, liver, or kidneys—were deprived of oxygen and essential nutrients. What might happen if this condition continued over a long period? It's almost as if you'd be "starving" these organs.

The problem is *we may have misalignments in our spine for years without ever realizing it.*

Chiropractors are known mostly for helping those with back and neck pains. But the benefits of the adjustments they do to the spine can go far beyond this, improving our nerves' ability to send essential signals to our various body parts. This can help prevent a variety of illnesses, such as heart disease, kidney failure, diabetes, poor circulation, and chronically poor sleep. Even some specific

146

dental problems can be helped through chiropractic care. According to an excellent chiropractor I know, Dr. Charlie Landgrebe, adjusting the mid- to upper-cervical spine and manually manipulating the surrounding muscles can relax the muscles in the face and neck and even relieve many of the symptoms of TMJ dysfunction (described in chapter 3).

If you are suffering from chronic fatigue, a chiropractor may be able to help. When is it time to visit one? Any time you decide that you could use a little more energy and vitality in your life.

## Air

Certainly, we take air for granted. We can't see it (hopefully), but we know it's there and take it into our lungs all day long with nary a thought.

The problem is that air just isn't what it once was. Now, oxygen is oxygen. The element itself isn't changing anytime soon. But the *amount* of oxygen in our air today *has* changed. It's been estimated that because of pollution, the air in some cities has 20 percent less oxygen than it once did. This means each time we inhale, we aren't taking in the same amount of oxygen that our ancestors were breathing in only a few generations ago. This should concern us. Oxygen plays a critical role in our health. It affects our blood circulation, our capability to assimilate nutrients, our ability to have a vigorous immune system, and our metabolism. It plays vital roles in rebuilding our bodies and assists our bodies in ridding themselves of waste and toxins. This all affects our energy level, which, as you know if you have been following so far, also affects our happiness.

We know that when we exercise hard, we soon find ourselves gasping for breath. But in ordinary life, could we be "gasping" for more oxygen too?

While our entire body depends on oxygen, the organ where we first notice a lack of it is our brain. If we don't get sufficient supplies of oxygen to our brain (say, after some kind of trauma), it can be permanently damaged. On a less severe scale, a drop in blood flow and oxygen can lead to lightheadedness. We momentarily can't think straight and may even lose balance.

It's clear that if the brain isn't getting everything it needs, it will be more challenging to have an abundance of vitality and joy. But ask yourself, other than moving to another part of the country (or another part of the world) where air is less polluted and oxygen more plentiful, is there really anything we can do?

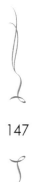

147

Actually, there is.

There is a medical approach to increasing your oxygen saturation that involves receiving pure oxygen under pressure. It's called *hyperbaric oxygen therapy*. You lie or sit in a chamber where oxygen is pumped in at about two times the normal air pressure. This intensely oxygenates your body, transporting it much more efficiently through the body's blood vessels.

You've probably already heard of such chambers being used to treat ocean divers who came up too rapidly (a condition known as the bends). Today, this technology has evolved and is being applied to many other conditions as well. Hyperbaric oxygen can be useful in treating severe burns, autism, certain brain injuries, diabetes, sports injuries, strokes, heart attacks, multiple sclerosis, Lyme disease, chronic fatigue syndrome, spinal cord injuries, certain wounds, chronic infections, migraines, poor skin, and even simple stress.

Obviously, the potential benefits are great. The biggest obstacles to its widespread use are the lack of treatment centers and the cost. Hour-long treatments can cost two hundred dollars, and you would most likely need daily treatments for ten days to two weeks to get the desired results. After that, any follow-up treatments would be much less frequent.

While home chambers do exist, they generally don't produce as much pressure and supply only about 75 percent oxygen. Still, that is nearly four times the oxygen levels you'd normally have, and the device—while expensive at about twenty thousand dollars—may be more economical in the long run, since you and anyone in your family could have access to it on a regular basis. If it truly can correct some chronic conditions that are otherwise incurable, it may not seem so expensive. I'm just letting you know that hyperbaric oxygen is available, and it's likely cheaper and more convenient than moving to some oxygen-rich tropical rainforest.

## Life Balance

In today's demanding times, it is becoming harder and harder to maintain equilibrium in our lives. Many of us focus too much on work. If we have children, we don't want the kids to be shortchanged either, and we strive to get them to all their soccer games, music lessons, tutoring, and art classes. It's a competitive world out there. Naturally, we all want to succeed, and we want our kids to succeed.

Yet, what's the point of competing—even if we win—if we aren't enjoying ourselves? Even though I have an intense focus on my dental practice, I endeavor to find time to relax and enjoy my family, as well as create time for hobbies.

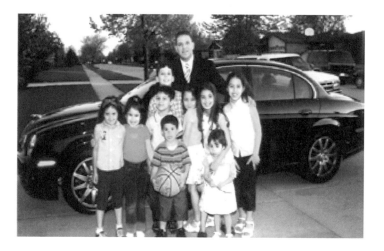

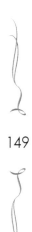

I love children. I love those I treat in my practice and the many children in my extended family. I couldn't wait to have kids of my own. These days, I truly love coming home to my beautiful wife and daughter. I just love walking through that door and hugging them, being with them. It brings me absolute and undeniable joy. Even though I have many demands on my time, I make sure I make time for all of us to be together.

I find other outlets where I can enjoy myself as well. I'm a scuba diver. I often go on dives off the coasts of Mexico, where I relish becoming immersed in schools of dazzlingly colorful fish.

I especially enjoy looking for fish that are hiding. (I suppose this is related to my passion for discovering patients' dental problems that others have missed.) It's like another world down there, magical and serene. I like it so much that I have big fish tanks in my office and my house.

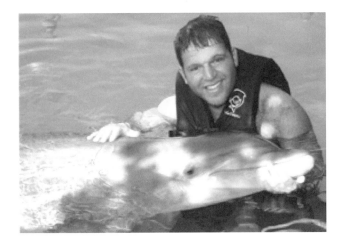

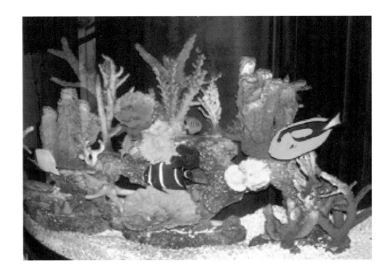

I also love riding horses, especially Arabians. They're so spunky and incredibly beautiful.

I even dabble in forensic dentistry. During my residency, I had the honor of being one of the few civilian residents chosen to participate in the United States Navy Forensic Team Course, and I became certified by the US Navy in forensic dentistry as well as oral pathology.

While I don't perform these functions like the detectives you see on the *CSI* shows, I continue going to the meetings and stay on top of the latest information. While some might think of this as more work, for me it is actually a great pleasure.

I recommend that everyone experience the true joy of finding balance in his or her life. It will most likely take some effort at first, as most good things do, especially as we change our habits. But it keeps us healthier and more joyful. As you've seen in this book, these two attributes are very much inter-

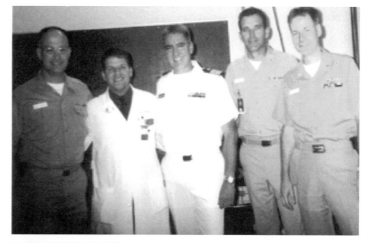

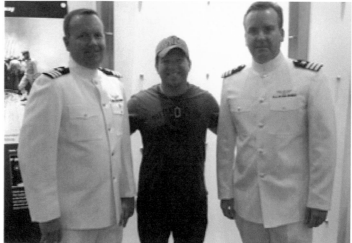

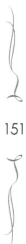

151

related. Honoring and taking true care of ourselves involves more than just having a mouth of healthy teeth and a robust body to go along with it. We should find time and activities that feed our souls and spirits, just as we seek out nourishing food, water, and air to feed our physical bodies.

This is my hope for all of you, and it is why I wanted to cover a variety of subjects be-

yond dentistry in this book. We are indeed the sum of our many parts, and something beyond even that.

Achieving balance in our lives, by tending to what's outside and what's inside, will go a long way toward helping us shine that happy, engaging, and irresistibly gorgeous *Chicago Smile*.

## ZACK ZAIBAK, MS, DDS

Dr. Zaibak is a licensed general dentist in the state of Illinois and one of Illinois' top practitioners of advanced cosmetic dentistry. Holding BS, BSD, DDS, and masters degrees, he has been honored by the Consumers Research Council of America as one of America's Top Dentists. He additionally has the latest advanced training and certification in Lumineers, Invisalign, and laser surgery. Today at his Chicago practice, Dr. Zaibak offers General Dentistry services as well as the Cosmetic Dentistry services for which he is renowned. Dr. Zaibak treats those needing severe dental reconstruction as well as those wishing to achieve a "Hollywood smile," including media personalities, models, and beautiful brides.

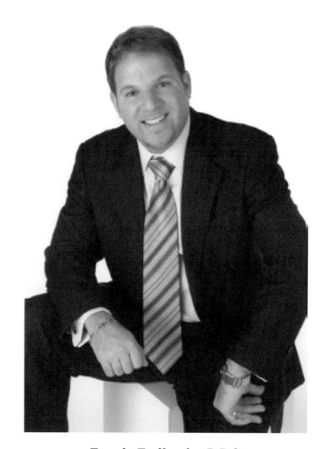

**Zack Zaibak, DDS**
**Zaibak Center for Dentistry**
**1.708.802.9600**
**www.drzaibak.com**

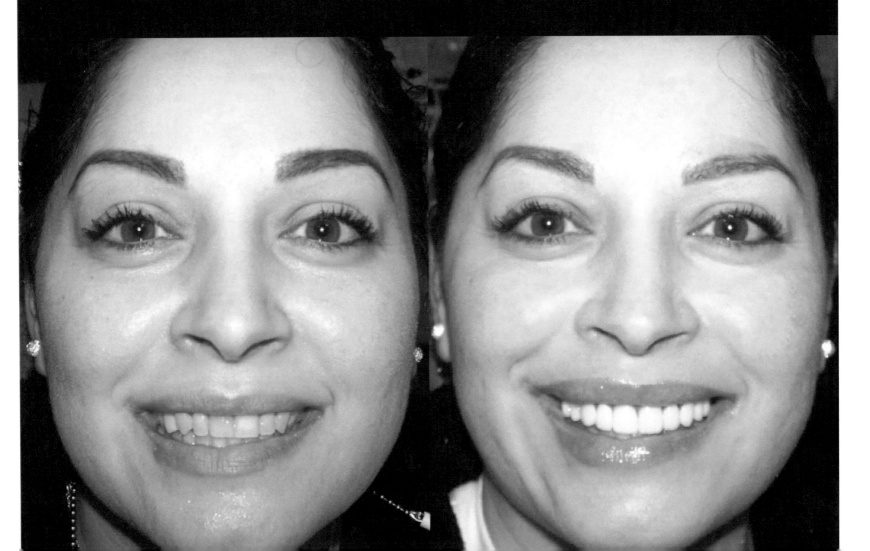

Smiles by Dr. Zack Zaibak

" GET YOUR SMILE BACK WITH DR. ZAIBAK "

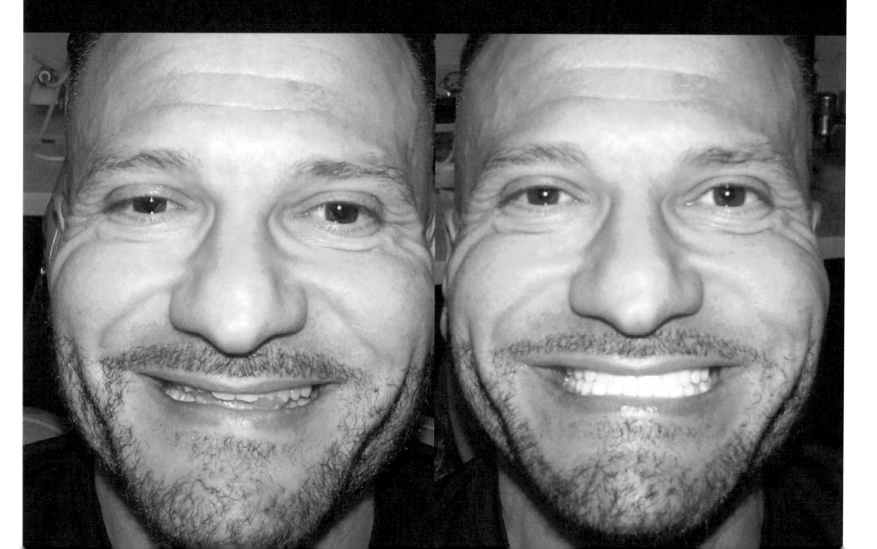

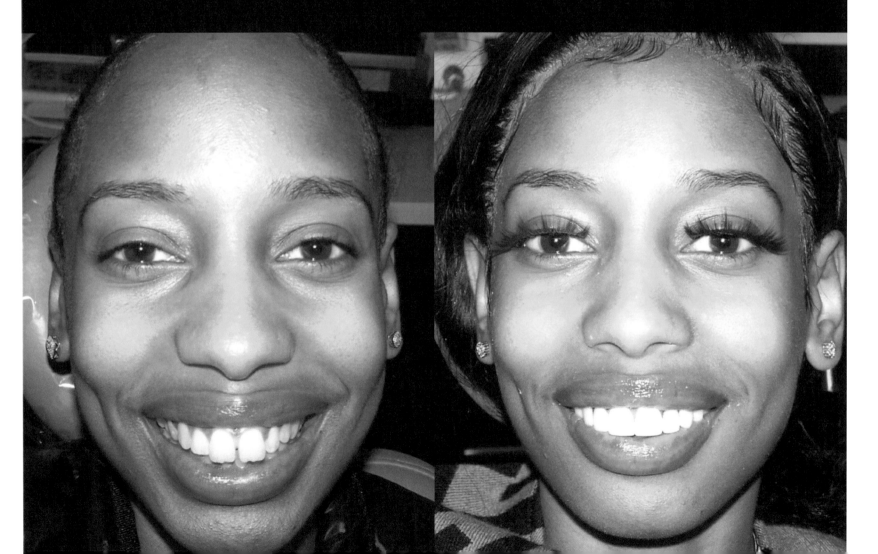

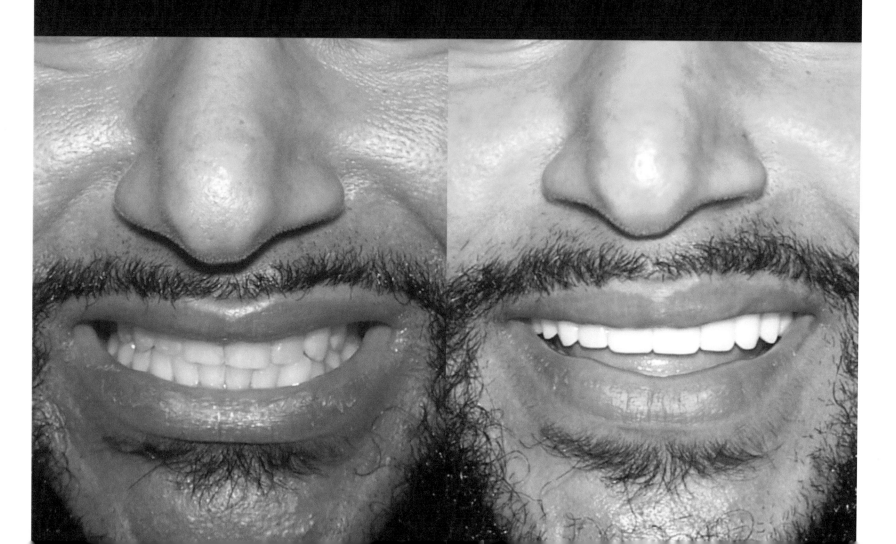

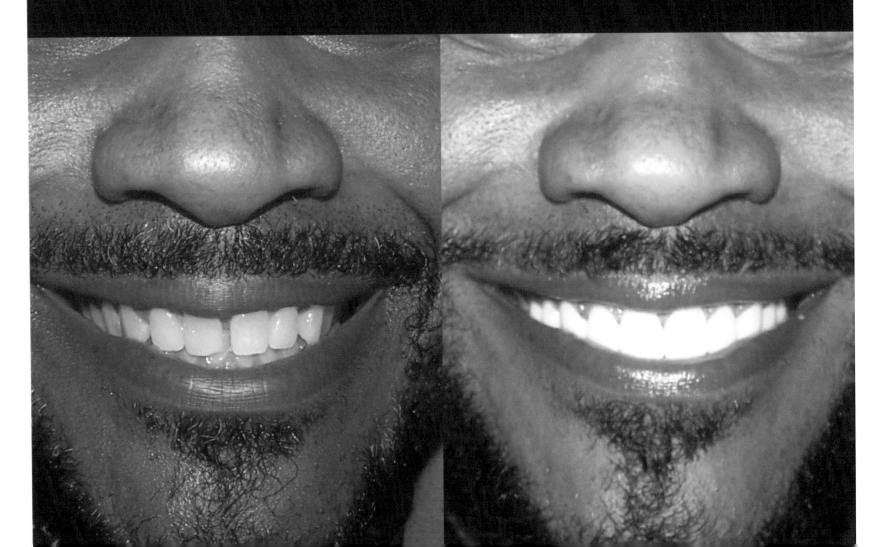

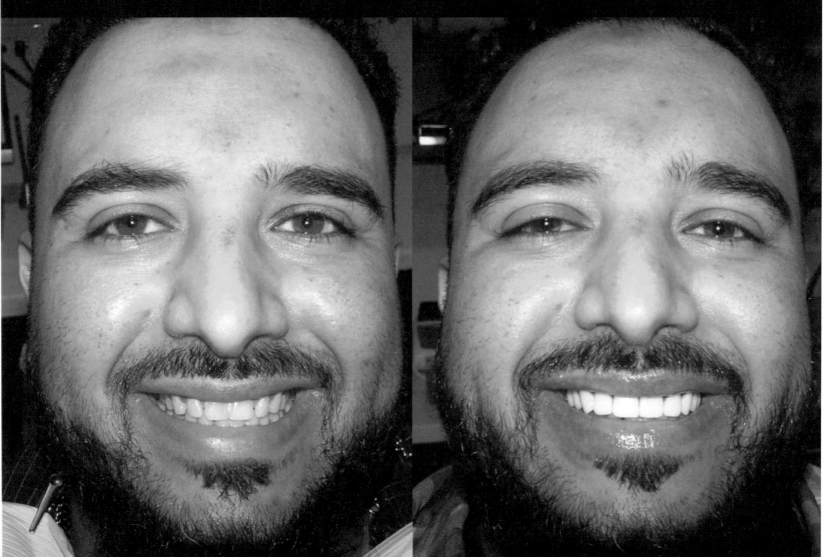

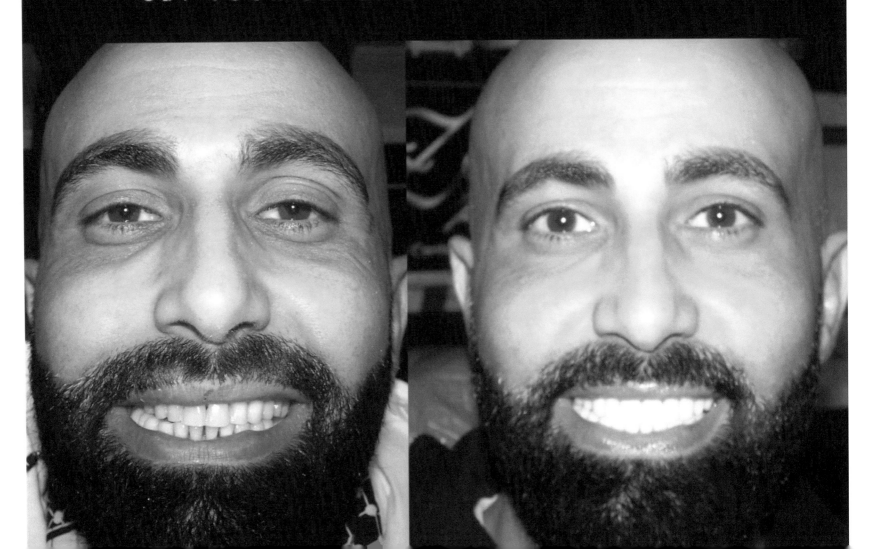

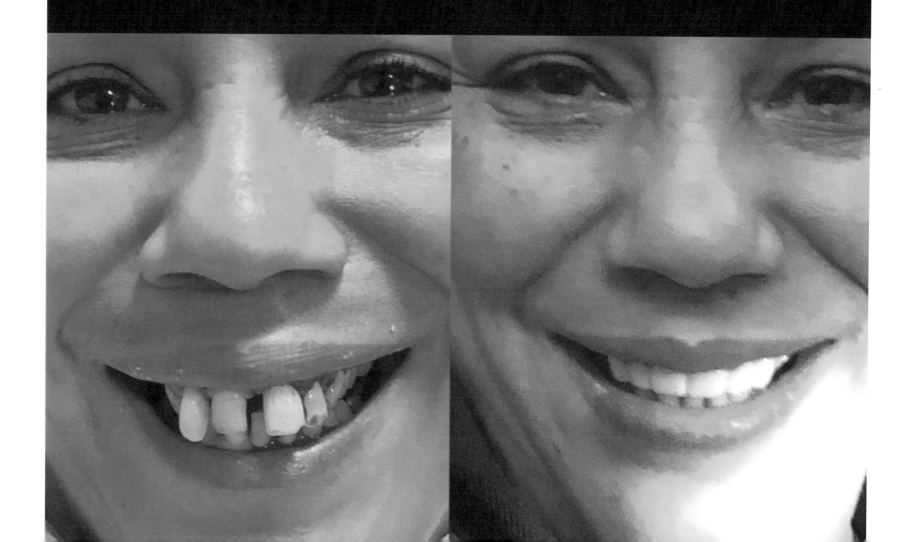

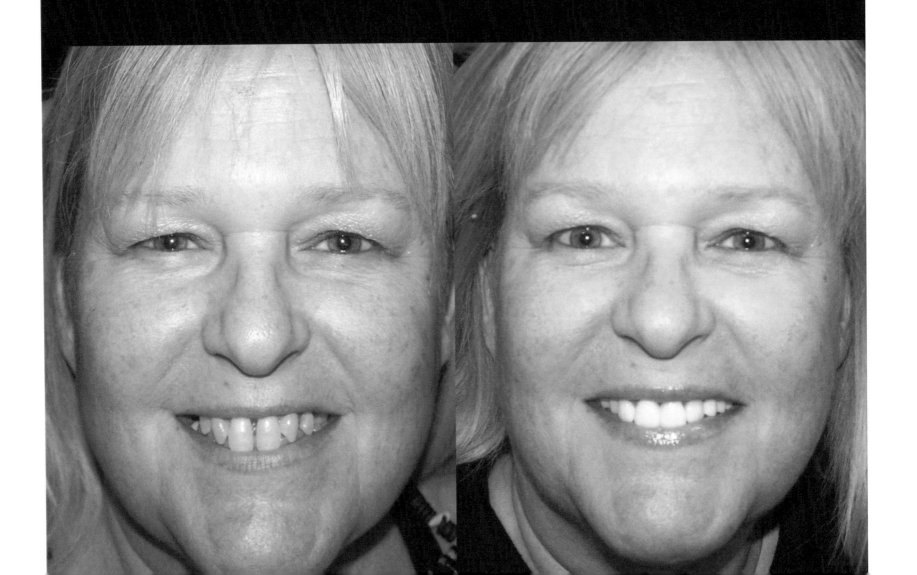

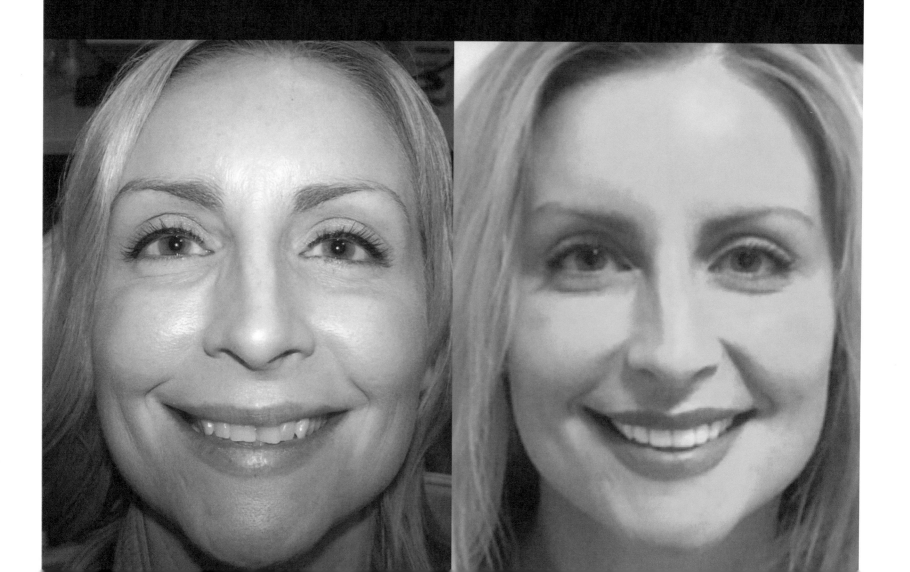

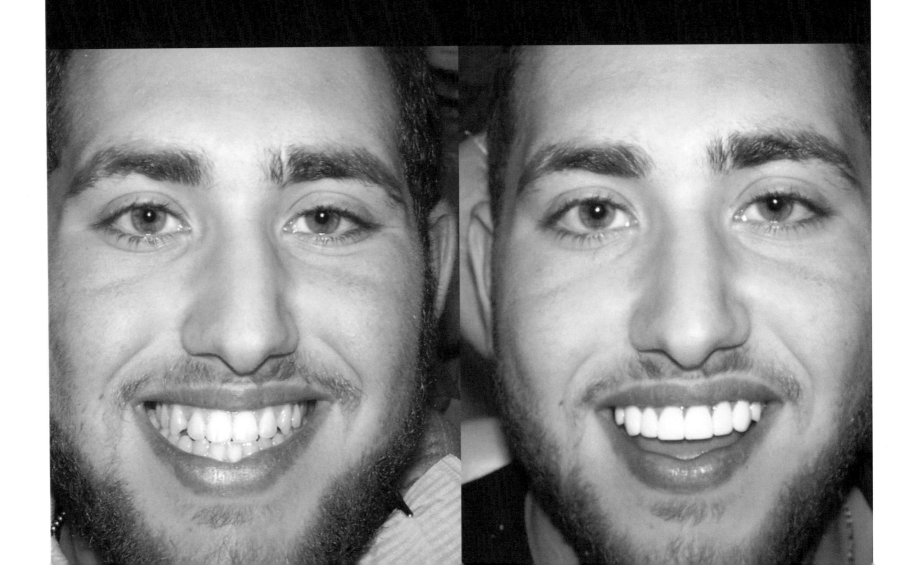

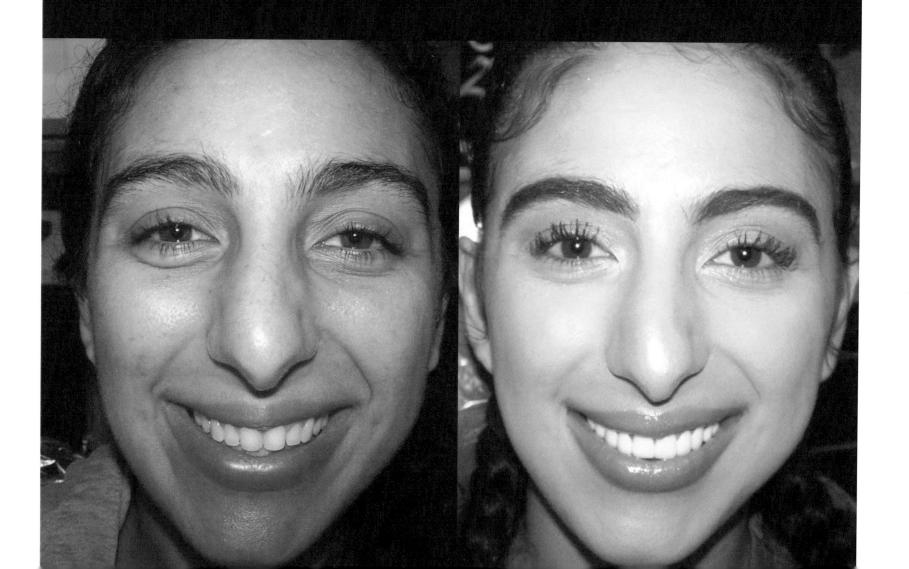

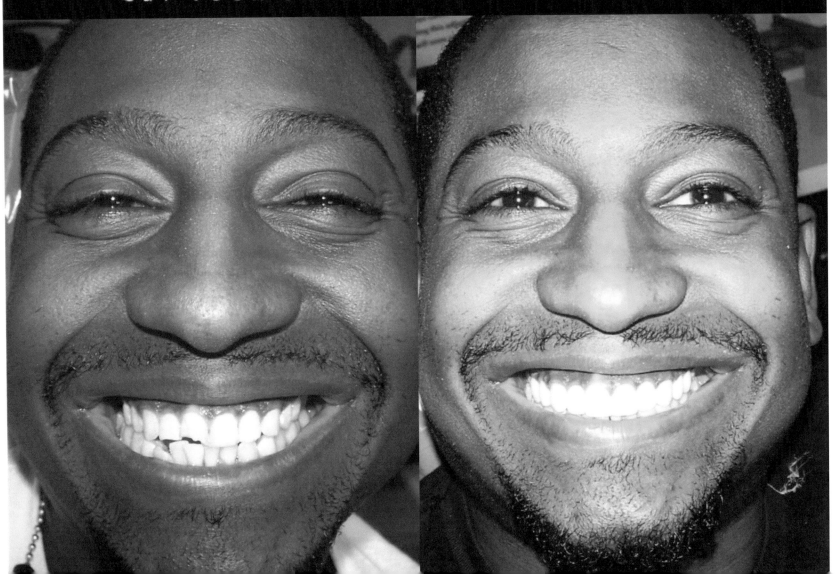

# Smiles by Dr. Zack Zaibak

" GET YOUR SMILE BACK WITH DR. ZAIBAK "

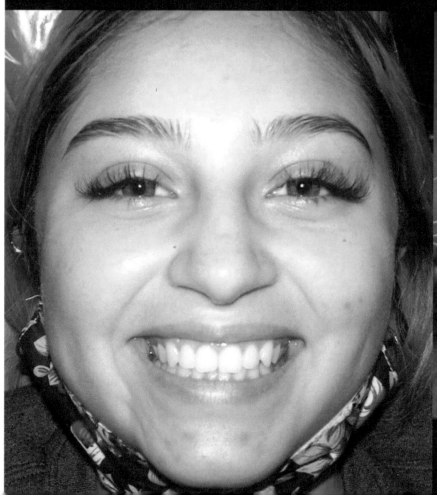
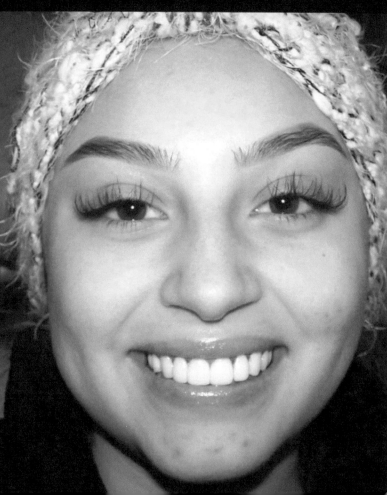

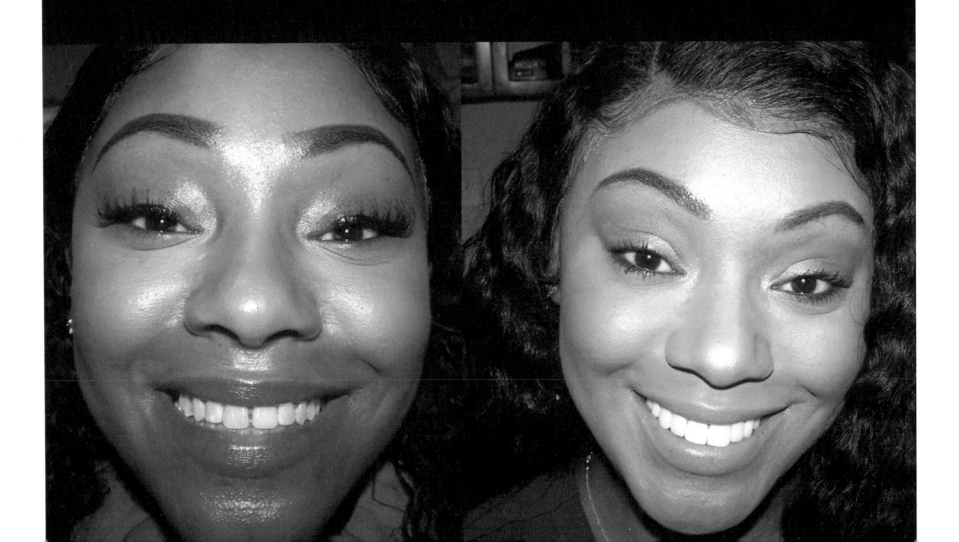